**Comisiwn
Bevan
Commission**

70 YEARS ON – WHAT NEXT?

Personal reflections on the NHS in Wales from the Bevan Commissioners

Edited by Dr Tom Powell & Hannah Scarbrough

D1334276

Published by Bevan Commission

70 YEARS ON – WHAT NEXT?

Personal reflections on the NHS in Wales from the Bevan Commissioners

Editorial material and organisation © 2018 Dr Tom Powell & Hannah Scarbrough

Published by Bevan Commission, www.bevancomission.org

Typesetting, production, and distribution by Wordcatcher Publishing, Cardiff, UK.
www.wordcatcher.com
02921 888321

Paperback ISBN: 978-1-912334-14-8
Ebook ISBN: 978-1-912334-07-0

Category: Health and Care

Table of Contents

The Bevan Commission

Comisiwn
Bevan
Commission

The Bevan Commission (hosted and supported by Swansea University) brings together a group of internationally renowned experts who provide independent, authoritative and expert advice on health and care nationally and internationally. The Bevan Commission identifies and shares best practice from healthcare systems around the world, building on the principles of the NHS as first articulated by Aneurin Bevan in 1948. The Commission provides informed and authoritative advice to improve health and care in Wales and its translation into practice. It helps to engage people within the system and those who use the system to innovate and try out and test the viability of their own ideas and new ways of working. The Bevan Commission believes that good health and care is everyone's responsibility; people, communities, local government, the workplace, and is not just the responsibility of the NHS.

The Bevan Commissioners

Professor Sir Mansel Aylward CB (Chair)
Professor Dame Sue Bailey OBE DBE
Nygaire Bevan
Professor Bim Bhowmick OBE DL
Professor Dame Carol Black DBE
Sir Ian Carruthers OBE
Mary Cowern
Professor Baroness Finlay of Llandaff
Professor Kamila Hawthorne MBE MD FRCGP FRCP FAcadMEd
    DRCOG DCH
Professor Trevor M. Jones CBE
Lt General (Ret) Louis Lillywhite CB MBE OStJ
Ann Lloyd CBE
Professor Ewan Macdonald OBE
Chris Martin
Professor Sir Michael Marmot MBBS MPH PhD FRCP FFPHM
    FMedSci FBA
Professor Sir Anthony Newman Taylor CBE
Dr Helen Paterson
Professor Phillip Routledge CBE
Fran Targett OBE
Professor Hywel Thomas CBE
Sir Paul Williams OBE KStJ DL
Professor John Wyn Owen CB

Current Special Advisors to the Commission

Current Special Advisors to the Bevan Commission: Professor Marcus
Longley, Professor Donna Mead OBE, Professor Marc Clement, and
Professor Ceri Phillips.

International Bevan Commissioners

Professor Donald Berwick (USA), Professor Gregor Coster (New Zealand), and Dr David Bratt (New Zealand).

Contact

All correspondence should be addressed to:

> The Bevan Commission,
> School of Management,
> Swansea University Bay Campus,
> Fabian Way,
> Swansea,
> SA1 8EN.

All reports produced by the Bevan Commission are published on the Commission website: www.bevancommission.org.

Find us on Twitter: @BevanCommission

Citations

Please cite the chapters in this book as: Chapter Author (2018) Chapter Title, in Powell, T. & Scarbrough, H. (Eds.), *70 Years On – What Next? Personal reflections on the NHS in Wales from the Bevan Commissioners.*

1

An international view of prudent healthcare

Donald M. Berwick KBE, MD, MPP, FRCP

Don is President Emeritus and Senior Fellow at the Institute for Healthcare Improvement (IHI), which he co-founded and led for 18 years. From July, 2010, to December, 2011, he served as President Obama's appointee as Administrator of the Centers for Medicare and Medicaid Services (CMS). He has served on the faculties of the Harvard Medical School and the Harvard School of Public Health, and is an elected member of the National Academy of Medicine.

I have had the great privilege of serving as a member and advisor to the Bevan Commission for over a decade, and this has allowed me to get to know at first hand the potential of Wales to develop a healthcare system that can be a worldwide model of an approach to improving the health and wellbeing of an entire population. The conditions in Wales are favourable for that vision. It is a country of the right size, with deep, historical investments in communitarian approaches to wellbeing, energised by an ethos of solidarity and a track record of entrepreneurship. Wales seems to understand as a culture that redesign and innovation can always lead to better outcomes.

The Prudent Healthcare framework is an especially important intellectual advance, not just for Wales but also for those of us around the world who strive for better health and healthcare. I want to explain why I feel so strongly about the promise of Prudent Healthcare as a model, and to encourage its careful study and explicit use throughout Wales from now on.

Those of us interested in quality, which is my career-long endeavour, know that the performance of a system is a product of its design. A mantra in the world of quality improvement, which I first heard from my friend and mentor, Dr. Paul Batalden, which has been called "The First Law of Improvement", is this: "Every system is perfectly designed to achieve exactly the results it gets." Design and redesign are the routes to improvement in any enterprise. If you want to improve, change the system.

We know that healthcare systems generally, both in Wales and worldwide, are not performing at the level needed by the people they serve. They don't reliably achieve the aims that society wishes for. And they are highly wasteful. That is not due to any defect in the motivation or intention of the healthcare workforce. It is due to failures of design of the healthcare system itself.

Healthcare around the world has historically been designed in a way that stacks the cards against success. By success I mean the Institute for Health Improvement Triple Aim: the simultaneous achievement of 1) better healthcare for individuals when they need care, 2) better health for populations and 3) lower per capita cost (so that health care is not wasting either public or private funds). The Triple Aim seeks both better care and better health at lower cost, through the engine of continuous improvement.

Prudent Healthcare, to me, is a remarkably efficient and compelling set of design principles that can guide the reconfiguration of care to better achieve the Triple Aim. All improvement is change, and Prudent Healthcare helps us know what to change.

Principle 1 – Achieve health and wellbeing with the public patients and professionals as equal partners through co-production

Co-production is not just a word; it is a basic, fundamental design idea for healthcare. Unlike a product such as a computer or television, healthcare is not something simply made by a producer and delivered to a customer. Instead, healthcare must inevitably be co-created by the patient and family with healthcare professionals. If we can really reorganise healthcare around the idea that the care and pursuit of wellbeing is always co-produced, always done jointly by the beneficiary and the person attempting to help, we will end up designing and operating a healthcare system with a completely new, more equitable balance of contribution. It would mean, arguably, a revolutionary change in the balance of power.

It's extremely exciting to see organisations move more towards such a new balance, where patients, families, communities, managers, and professionals are working together to create better health and better health care. The modern digital world of telemedicine and telehealth helps cross old boundaries and open new ways for us to use knowledge together to achieve better health and wellbeing.

Principle 2 – Care for those with the greatest need first, making the most effective use of all skills and resources

The second principle is a moral principle: help those first who most need the help. Like co-production, this is a fundamental design idea for healthcare. It makes it clear that we need to configure resource investments, the use of capital, and the competence of both the public and professionals around the idea that our duties begin (though they do not end) with helping the most vulnerable people in our societies.

If we are to make the most effective use of all skills and resources, healthcare should incorporate and embrace community-based resources and the energies of entire populations to help meet the needs of the most vulnerable first. Indeed, the same idea – to use the abundance around us – applies equally to the care of everyone. This design principle widens the concept of healthcare itself, bringing effort and attention far outside the boundaries of the traditional institutions, professions, and disciplines of healthcare to date. It implies new alliances, unprecedented cooperation, and reallocation of resources.

Principle 3 – Do only what is needed, no more and no less, and do no harm

The third principle requires that we ask very hard questions in healthcare about what really helps and what does not help and where we may actually be causing harm. The legacy designs in healthcare systems often trap us all, like a gerbil in a gerbil cage, running and running, doing more and more things without pausing and asking why? When are we truly using resources and time in ways that actually help people, and when are we simply wasting time, money, supplies, and spirit? A sophisticated inquiry and trusting dialogue between the public and professionals around what really does help and what does not help will lead to healthcare that is far more sustainable, and less wasteful of the talents and energies of patients, families, communities and professionals.

If we focus on patient safety, we will be following a trail already blazed in Wales with the 1,000 Lives Campaign, which emphasises the avoidance of injuries that come from errors, poor designs, and miscalculations. A focus on safety truly places the patient at the centre. Prudent Healthcare could help make Welsh care nothing less than the safest in the world.

Principle 4 – Reduce inappropriate variation using evidence-based practices consistently and transparently

The fourth principle emphasises that healthcare at its best is informed by the scientific method. That principle does not imply any important loss of professional autonomy; it speaks rather to the gaining of professional reliability. It avows that applying evidence-based practices consistently and transparently is an important design rule for the healthcare systems of the future, which honours, rather than constrains, the intent of the healthcare workforce. The commitment to evidence-based care demands that we continually learn from each other to seek and find what really is best. It embraces transparency, and encourages all to discover and learn from the variations among us – to be able to find out that hospital A is doing better than hospital B, and then to illuminate why and how, to the benefit of all. It discourages any reliance on blame, exhortation, and even incentive, and it encourages and celebrates joint and mutual learning.

A commitment to evidence, properly implemented, does not forge handcuffs. It does not mean that physicians, surgeons, nurses, pharmacists and therapists stop using their minds and intuitions. It is crucial to preserve the opportunities for clinicians to adjust care continually at the 'sharp end', so that intelligent, alert people can always do the right thing, even when it sometimes strays from the general standard. But the basic design principle of reducing inappropriate variation – the random variation that is not cognizant of the underlying science – is a value at the heart of the Prudent Healthcare framework.

In summary

Wales can be a learning nation. For Wales, and for the world, that is an exciting vision. The four principles of Prudent Healthcare together compose one of the richest frameworks I have encountered in helping to define the healthcare that is capable of achieving the Triple Aim, and continually improving. My hope and plea for Wales is to achieve continually better care, better health, and lower cost, not through the historic system and not through technically bankrupt approaches of mere exhortation, requirement, and incentive, but rather through the design and embrace of a new healthcare system, all together, conceived and developed in Wales, by Wales, and for Wales. The changes will not come easily, and the commitment at the start to shared study, understanding, and embrace of each and all of the principles of Prudent Healthcare will be essential for success. But I firmly believe that those who seek clear guidance for building that new structure for Triple Aim health and care, with renewed joy for the workforce, will find none better than that offered by Prudent Healthcare – a Welsh gift to the world.

2

Back to the future, a system fit for the future

Helen Howson

Helen is the Director of the Bevan Commission and the Bevan Commission Academy. She has played a lead role in the development of the Commissions work and particularly Prudent Healthcare. Helen was instrumental in establishing the Bevan Academy, Bevan Innovators and Innovation Hub programmes, helping to drive its thinking into practice. She was previously a Public Health Consultant with Public Health Wales, leading a major Ministerial review of health improvement interventions across Wales. Prior to this Helen held a number of senior positions within Welsh Government Health Policy and Strategy, latterly heading up the Primary and Community Health Strategy Unit. Helen has worked as an advisor with the World Health Organisation and also advised Russian, Spanish, New Zealand and other Governments on health policy. Helen taught for a number of years on the WHO masters at Karolinska University in Sweden and at Bristol University as Director of a post-graduate Leadership programme for clinicians.

*Insanity is doing the same thing over and over again
and expecting different results.*

Albert Einstein

Why change?

Stephen Hawking (2017) in his *Theory of the NHS* used both his personal experiences and his scientific skills to reinforce the case for a National Health System as the most humane system in which all people are provided for equally, based upon their individual needs and without regards for their personal circumstances, their ability to pay, whether young or old. He believed that the most efficient way to provide good healthcare was for services to be publicly funded and publicly run whilst recognising the need to find ways in which health and the care system can provide care most efficiently without waste of labour or resources.

The NHS was designed 70 years ago in a time and for a need which is very different to what we have today. We have considerably different societal and heath and care needs, based largely upon the success of the NHS in helping people to live longer, but also upon the impact of the lifestyles that have evolved during that time

The society in which we live now is also very different. The use of technology in our everyday lives has seen an unprecedented growth. This can be seen in the use of technology whether mobile phones, the use of computers and the impact of social media, alongside the incredible developments made in the management and treatment of illness, disease and disability. These driving forces in the life science industry will impact upon both the quality and quantity of our lives.

As health consumers, we will be exposed to possibilities within a complex national health system which still has to deal with the day to day issues of growing demand, limited resources and managing consumer and professional expectations. We need to change to ensure we are making the very most of the assets we have around us as well as ensuring that we are able and fit for what the future might bring. The Bevan Commission's prudent approach to health aims to try to help achieve this, using its four principles (Bevan Commission, 2015) to help guide its approach and its delivery in practice.

So why don't we change?

The barriers to change are well known (Bevan Commission, 2016) and in essence this is primarily about people and the complexity of human behaviour and the large systems and leadership of the organisations within which they work. Some people like change, some do not, some are unsettled or even fear change and some are not even aware of the need to change or are not empowered to tackle the change as they see is needed.

It is also about how we create the climate to enable change to be an implicit part of everyday life. Creating a culture for change can be as basic as making sure that people know why change is needed, involving them in helping to find solutions and demonstrating the impact that this will have by improving care. Finding time to think about things differently is crucial, otherwise it is easy to keep doing the same things in the same way – we sometimes do the same things even better which can make the case for change even harder.

As healthcare becomes increasingly complex, whether through technology, new drugs or treatments, the system itself or the complexity of problems being presented, the approach to ensure quality and consistency tends to be tighter control, top down directives and more and more targets.

So how do we change?

*We can't solve todays problems using the
same thinking that created them.*

Albert Einstein

Whilst we have seen some incremental changes and improvements across the NHS, often supported by improvement thinking and methodologies, health and care leaders nationally and globally have begun to challenge such traditional approaches to change. There is a growing recognition that small incremental changes to existing models of care based upon traditional ways of thinking is no longer viable to meet future health and care needs and ensure the future sustainability of the NHS.

The Parliamentary Review into Health and Social Care in Wales (2018) called for 'revolution not evolution' and a new system of care where change is significantly accelerated 'unless faster, more widespread progress can be unlocked, access to and the quality of services will decline in the face of the predictable pressures'.

The review recognised the assets and power of service users and communities in driving change, along with the ability of the workforce to test and learn what works and to accelerate change and innovation. The Review also recognised that staff are sometimes doing so against the tide and identified the need for leaders to take 'bold decisions', advocating for increased capacity at a national level to drive transformation and stronger leadership nationally, regionally and locally.

The National Improvement Body for the NHS in England has also recognised the need for radical change in health and care systems. We live in a world where the 'power of hierarchy is diminishing' and that change is happening faster and becoming more disruptive (Bevan & Fairman, 2017). A better balance is suggested between existing approaches with new thinking and practice in leading change. From one based predominantly on transactional processes of authority and hierarchy, to one of transformation in which connection and the ability to influence through networks dominates.

The Chartered Institute for Personnel and Development report on landing transformational change (CIPD, 2014), identifies the need for transformational change in the following three areas - techniques to design change, build understanding and manage change:

- The design of transformational change requires senior executives to be adept at reading and rewriting their context, aligning strategy and culture, and delivering radical change opportunistically.
- Techniques that can build understanding include the use of ambiguity and purposeful instability; narratives, storytelling and conversations; and physical representation, metaphors and play.
- Management of the process requires relational leadership, building trust, voice and dialogue, and maintaining energy and momentum.

However, the capability to translate this thinking into action seems to be a consistent problem across many countries, so just how do we make the transformational changes needed?

Leading and leaders for change

Leaders and leadership are crucial to this in setting the tone, climate and culture to encourage and support it. In 2014 Michael West said 'collective and inclusive NHS leadership is the only way forward "and justified this by saying – traditional top down approaches had limitations, not sufficient to face the challenges we have today, or indeed in the future' (West, 2014). Current leaders have many challenges, a huge portfolio and they cannot focus on everything. Therefore, the very traditional top down leadership role will need to change to one of distributive, collective and collaborative leadership in which all staff are encouraged to adopt leadership roles and with that take joint responsibility for improving the quality of care and health outcomes.

Collaboration, trust and empowering people to do what is right for the patient is essential. It involves driving innovation and supporting a wider learning environment in which risks are managed and shared. We may not get it right in the first instance but we need to trust colleagues to have a go and to effectively manage that risk.

The Bevan Commission has recognised the importance of collective and collaborative leadership as a fundamental ingredient in helping to transform health and care in Wales for some time. This, alongside innovation and social movements for change form the core elements underpinning its Bevan Academy and Bevan Innovators programme which aims to help translate its thinking into practice.

Bevan Academy and Bevan Innovators; driving change

The Bevan Commission has over the last 5 years given considerable thought to the need to lead and drive transformational change. In recognition of this the Commission set up the Bevan Academy to help translate its thinking into practice. It recognised from the outset that this could only be effectively achieved by engaging people who work in the system and also those who use the system. Finding and developing strong courageous leaders at all levels with great ideas, who were innovative, creative and passionate about being part of driving these ideas forward, formed the core of the Bevan Innovators' programme.

To help expedite change and try out and test new ideas we created Bevan Innovators which included; Bevan Exemplars (staff from within the NHS), Bevan Fellows (early career clinicians) and Bevan Advocates (members of the public passionate about the sustainability of the NHS). With the Bevan Exemplars we asked people across the NHS at all levels, 'have you got some ideas? – Are they prudent and would you like to work with us to try out and test them?' We gave them 12 months and a programme of support which they co designed based upon what they felt they needed i.e. designed for them by them.

We had some surprising results and met some fascinating people who might otherwise have remained one of 80,000 employees within the system. We gave them: support, kudos, credibility and coverage, should things go array – they gave us: energy, enthusiasm, ideas and passion for a sustainable and innovative social movement for change. The independent evaluation of the first cohort of exemplars (Rich. 2017) indicated that 70% were successful contrary to other recent studies by Ham et al. (2016) which indicated that innovation was more likely to be in the region of 30% successful. Further evaluation has reaffirmed this for cohort 2 and identified additional benefits in terms of other spin off ideas as well as building confidence, competence and empowered leaders for the future.

As an NHS we need to get better at empowering and trusting our staff and our patients to look for those opportunities to do better things and be part of creating better outcomes and personal experiences. They are out there at the coal front and they see, hear and know what needs to be done to make things better and, in some cases, it can be a matter of asking them what works rather than telling them what to do. We need to be able to give them the opportunity to do so by building their own resilience within a supportive and sustainable environment.

We need to continually learn from each other, maximising the skills, assets and opportunities that we have amongst our 80,000 strong workforce across NHS Wales as well as those who use our services daily. We should be enabling and empowering people to be part of the solutions using and applying their great ideas and the opportunities that they present to us. We should seek to develop more creative, confident and competent organisations, capable of leading the transformational changes needed so that we have a health and care system that is fit for the future.

Learning from our learning; helping making it happen in practice

We have had the privilege to work with over 120 remarkable individuals across NHS Wales during the past 3 years. They have demonstrated greater confidence and know how in their work as well as a greater sense of self belief and confidence whilst working with us. The following sets out some of the important components that we have identified which will help ensure we have a better chance of translating ideas into practice;

- **New thinking** – for an organisation to drive transformational change it will need to think differently and be receptive to fundamental change. As long as ideas remain 'projects' or initiatives on the periphery, then that is where they will remain.
- **Honesty and openness** – is essential to help maximise ideas and to create a climate of trust should things not succeed.
- **Commitment** – there is no point in putting pen to paper, writing edicts and strap lines if there is no commitment to see things through. This is a journey of discovery; it is unpredictable and everyone should accept this for the long term.
- **Creating a climate for change** – moving from transactional to transformational processes where connections, networks and relationships are equally important rather than just traditional top down hierarchies. Empowering and trusting people to use their judgement to help drive the changes across and between organisations.
- **Building upon what we have** – a plethora of great ideas, passion and commitment already exists within staff and patients. Using levers and incentives will help find these, building upon schemes such as the Bevan Exemplars and Advocates and other developments.
- **A platform to try out and test** – create an environment in which people are expected continually to find new and better ways of working so that it is everyone's business not just the few. Find ways to make it easier and more open for staff – giving them headroom to think, taking their ideas seriously and bringing people together.
- **Support and encouragement** – sometimes people need a little help or moral support to get through barriers or just advice on how best to take things next – other support such as training or access to other expertise or views can help.

- **Recognising and rewarding success** – many people are self-motivated and identify and drive change because they are passionate about making things better. Simple rewards, recognition and acknowledgement goes a long way in boosting morale and confidence.
- **Sharing, adapting and adopting** – finding and developing new ideas can be relatively simple compared to the widespread adoption. Using the passion of the people who developed it to encourage others to adopt can help and avoids being driven from top down.

It is clear that we have a strong and overriding consensus on the need for change and for that change to be radical and imminent. There is also acceptance of the need for more fundamental change based upon transformational approaches using the skills and networks we already have within our staff and patients.

We should therefore get on and do something based upon what we know to date, rather than wait for the perfect formulae and learn by doing – not by pontificating or waiting for policies or legislation to work.

Using the skills and knowledge of people in the system and those who use the system is as yet relatively untapped. Changing the language to one which asks clinicians what works rather than telling them what to do may be part of the solution and part of re balancing the locus of control.

From what we have seen to date from our Bevan Exemplars, we should build on this urgently, refining and learning as we go, creating a social movement for change from inside and outside the NHS and tapping in to the passion and power of people.

References

Bevan Commission. (2015). Prudent Health Principles.

Bevan Commission. (2016). The Barriers and Enablers to Change.

Bevan, H. & Fairman, S. (2017) The new era of thinking and practice in change and transformation, NHSIQ.

CIPD. (2014) Landing Transformational Change.

Ham, C., Bewick, D. & Dixon, J. (2016) Improving quality in the English NHS A strategy for action. Kings Fund.

Hawking, S. (2017) Theory of the NHS. Journal of the Royal Society of Medicine. 2017. Vol. 110 (12) 460-473.

Parliamentary Review into Health and Social Care. (2018) Welsh Government.

Rich, N. (2017) Evaluation of the Bevan Innovators Exemplar Programme Cohort One. Bevan Commission, Swansea, UK ISBN 978-1-912334-00-1.

West, M. (2014) Collective and Collaborative Leadership. Kings Fund.

3

Aneurin Bevan and the origins of the NHS

Professor Sir Antony Newman Taylor CBE

Sir Anthony is the President's Envoy for Health, Imperial College and Director of Research and Development, National Heart and Lung Institute, Imperial College. He was Principal of the Faculty of Medicine at Imperial College between 2010 and 2012, having previously held the position of Deputy Principal for the Faculty since 2008 and Head of the National Heart and Lung Institute between 2006 and 2008. He is currently Chairman of the Health and Safety Executive Workplace Health Expert Committee, Chairman of the Colt Foundation, Chairman of the Independent Medical Expert Group of the Armed Forces Compensation Scheme (AFCS) for Ministry of Defence, a Trustee of the Rayne Foundation and a Member of the Advisory Board, Royal British Legion Centre for Blast Injury Studies (CBIS), Imperial College.

> *No society can legitimately call itself civilised if a sick*
> *person is denied medical aid because of lack of means.*

Aneurin Bevan, *In Place of Fear*

The National Health Service is the enduring legacy of the implementation of the Beveridge Report recommendations by the 1945-50 Labour government, arguably the most radical UK government in the 20th century. Aneurin Bevan, Minister of Health is rightly recognised, and by many revered, as the founder of the NHS. But the foundations on which his achievement was built go back to the turn of the century, some 50 years before the 1948 Act that brought the NHS into being.

The concept of provision by the state of healthcare was first considered in the aftermath of the Boer War, with the recognition that the health of a significant proportion of the adult population was too poor for them to be fit for military recruitment. For instance, White, using the records of the Royal Army Medical Corps reported that, "In the Manchester district 11,000 men offered themselves for war service between the outbreak of hostilities in October 1899 and July 1900. Of this number 8,000 were found to be physically unfit to carry a rifle and stand the fatigues of discipline. Of the 3,000 who were accepted only 1,200 attained the moderate standard of muscular power and chest measurement required by the military authorities. In other words, two out of every three men willing to bear arms in the Manchester district are virtually invalids." In large part this was a reflection of the poverty and poor nutrition of many of those living and working in UK cities.

Further evidence of this came from the findings of two influential surveys at the turn of the century. Charles Booth investigated the prevalence of poverty in London and Seebohm Rowntree in York. Both concluded that about ⅓ of the population of these cities lived at some time during their lives below the poverty line. The impact of these reports led to the Tory government in 1905 setting up a Royal Commission on the Poor Laws and Relief of Distress, which reported in 1909. Beatrice Webb, a member of the Commission who disagreed fundamentally with the conclusions of the main report, wrote the *Minority Report*, calling for greater government intervention, with the need for an integrated system of relief that covered health and employment. She was the first to propose a 'public' or 'state' medical service in which, "Neither the promptitude nor the efficiency of the medical treatment (was) in any way limited by considerations of whether the patient can or should repay its cost". Jose Harris in his biography of William Beveridge, said that "in historical accounts of modern social policy, the Royal Commission and in particular its famous *Minority Report* has often been twinned with the Beveridge Plan of 1942 as one of the two most seminal enquiries into the working of British social policy in the last 100 years".

In 1906, some three years before the publication of the Royal Commission report, the Liberals were returned to government. The Chancellor, David Lloyd George, in 1911 introduced the National Insurance Act, which for the first time provided health insurance for wage earners, between the ages of 16 and 70, earning less than £160 per year. Lloyd George's slogan of 'ninepence for fourpence' encapsulated the contribution of 4d for male (3d for female) employees, 3d from the employer and 2d from the state. Lloyd George became known as Lord George, because only a Lord could afford to be so generous. The benefits for insured workers included sick pay for up to 26 weeks and treatment from a doctor on a government list of approved practitioners, who would receive a set fee for the service. Men could also claim a maternity allowance for the cost of an attendant for their wife during childbirth. Some 2.25 million signed on and a large amount of previously unrecognised ill health came to light. However, the 1911 National Insurance Act excluded hospital care and many people, including non-working wives and the children of those insured as well as higher income workers and many of the elderly.

Aneurin Bevan, who was born in 1897, grew up in Tredegar in South Wales during the early years of the 20th century. The son of a miner, he left school aged 13 to work with his father in Ty Tryst Colliery. In common with many coalfields in South Wales, Tredegar had founded a Workmen's Medical

Aid Society. By 1920 the Tredegar Workmen's Medical Aid Society provided the services of five doctors, one surgeon, two pharmacists, a physiotherapist, a dentist and a district nurse, for roughly 95% of the local population. The value of a universal healthcare service available to all was certainly influenced by his experience in Tredegar. As Bevan later wrote, "The essence of a satisfactory health service is that the rich and the poor are treated alike and poverty is not a disability and wealth not an advantage."

During the inter-war years, state provision of healthcare in the United Kingdom remained essentially unchanged from the Lloyd George Act in 1911, despite the provision of a comprehensive state health service becoming Labour party policy in 1934.

Hospital care remained outside the Act and before 1939 hospital services were provided by voluntary and municipal hospitals. The voluntary hospitals included the London teaching and post graduate hospitals, originally dependent on voluntary contributions, but increasingly dependent on fee paying patients. Consultants had honorary unpaid appointments so that the voluntary hospitals were, and therefore specialist care was, concentrated where private patients resided, in the more prosperous parts of the country. Many of the municipal hospitals had been formed as part of the 1834 workhouse scheme and run by local authorities. They were generally considered the poor cousins of the voluntary hospitals, with surgery and anaesthesia provided in many by local GPs.

By 1939 both the voluntary hospitals and the municipal hospitals were in severe financial difficulties. The physical condition of many was poor, several were bankrupt and the quality of service provision, particularly out of main urban areas, often dire.

The war brought important changes. Surveys in 1937 and 1938 had pointed to the deficiencies of hospital services in England and fear of the consequences of the Blitz led to the creation of the Emergency Medical Service (EMS) in which, by late 1939, the government had invested in tens of thousands of additional beds, nearly 1,000 new operating theatres and equipment, as well as the creation of a national transfusion service. The EMS steadily increased the number of those eligible for treatment, so that by the end of the war a significant proportion of the population was included in a free hospital service run by the Ministry of Health.

In his 1942 report Beveridge identified Disease as one of the 5 giants that stood on the road to post war reconstruction, together with Want, Ignorance, Squalor and Idleness. He proposed a radically changed system of social security, based on contributory payments: "Benefit in return for contributions". To achieve this, he identified three assumptions as pre-requisites for his recommendations for a modernised system of social security.

Allowances of 8 shillings per week for the upkeep of children to the end of their full time compulsory education. Seebohm Rowntree had identified that, after unemployment, family size was the major reason for poverty and Beveridge saw child allowance as necessary as part of his attack on poverty.

Free and universal health service. Beveridge appreciated that it was in the state's interest to provide free health care, including hospital inpatient treatment, both to prevent ill health and to keep those claiming sickness benefit to a minimum.

Economic policies which prevented mass unemployment. Beveridge recognised that a benefit system dependent on flat rate contributions would collapse with a sustained period of high unemployment.

Public reception of the Beveridge report was extremely favourable, forcing the Wartime Coalition Government to accept the recommendations, at least in principle. Sales of the report exceeded any HMSO publication until Lord Denning's report into the Profumo affair. The timing of the report was fortunate, following shortly after Montgomery's victory at El Alamein, in Churchill's words, "the end of the beginning". Plans for post war reconstruction were becoming a reality. Following the Beveridge Report proposals were formulated by the Coalition Government in early 1944 in a White Paper entitled *A National Health Service.*

The 1944 White Paper proposed a 'comprehensive' health care service, free at the point of use, funded out of taxation. The proposals for hospital services were that the municipal hospitals should be run by boards of grouped local authorities, while the voluntary hospitals should be free to make contracts with the boards for 'the performance of agreed services'.

While the principles of a comprehensive national health service free at the point of use and funded out of taxation had been enunciated in the 1944 White Paper, how such a service might be delivered was far from clear. Bevan's achievement and legacy were the delivery of a workable and enduring service within three years of entering office. He was a formidable and effective politician, described as "an artist in the use of power". It was typical that his first decision on entering the Ministry in 1945 was to insist on the removal of the armchair in the Minister's office: "This won't do. It drains all the blood from the head and explains a lot about my predecessors!"

In setting up the NHS, Bevan faced two important problems: the organisation of the hospital service and payment of hospital consultants; and the organisation and basis for payment of general practitioners. He recognised immediately the weaknesses in the proposals in the 1944 White Paper for hospitals, which were fragmented, and unworkable, the consequence of many compromises with the medical profession. In a master-stroke he decided to take all the hospitals – both voluntary and municipal – into public ownership. This was not without opposition in the Cabinet, notably from Herbert Morrison, who had made his name before the war as leader of the London County Council. Morrison was concerned that removing responsibility for hospitals from local authorities would seriously diminish their influence. Bevan proposed that the hospitals be accountable to regional health boards, responsible to the Minister. In another masterstroke, he made friends with the Presidents of the three main Royal Colleges: of Physicians, of Surgeons and of Obstetricians and Gynaecologists, who represented the senior hospital consultants. Of these, the President of the Royal College of Physicians, Lord Moran, widely known as Corkscrew Charlie, Winston Churchill's personal physician, was the most important. To achieve his goal of securing the support of the hospital consultants, Bevan was prepared to compromise on several fronts. While salaried, hospital consultants would be allowed to retain private beds in NHS hospitals, to have part time appointments to allow time for private practice and be eligible for additional payments, 'merit awards', whose award, in the first instance, was decided by Moran and his colleagues. He was later to say, "I stuffed their mouths with gold". But he achieved their support and backing.

Although both the hospital consultants and the GPs were officially represented by the British Medical Association (BMA), Bevan had divided the consultants from the GPs. The BMA in their negotiations with Bevan essentially now represented the interests of GPs. The BMA was violently opposed to the introduction of a national health service, fearing that a salaried service would make civil servants of doctors, who would lose their clinical freedom and freedom of speech. Between 1946 and July 1948, the vesting date for the NHS, Bevan persisted with difficult and often fractious negotiations with the BMA. By early 1948, the BMA, or at least its GP members, were persuaded that a full time salaried GP service with loss of clinical freedom and the right of patients to choose their GP was not Bevan's intention. By vesting day, July 5, 1948, 90% of GPs in England had enrolled in the NHS and 75% (reaching 97% a few months later) of patients had put their names on GPs lists. It was a remarkable triumph for Bevan.

Two others of Bevan's contemporaries in government and a third outside government also deserve recognition for the critical part they played in the birth of the NHS: the Prime Minister, Clement Attlee, the Chancellor of the Exchequer, Hugh Dalton, and John Maynard Keynes. Attlee can lay claim to be England's greatest peacetime prime minister in the 20th century. His choice of Bevan, no friend of his during the Wartime Coalition, as Minister of Health was inspired. Throughout the difficult period of negotiations with the BMA, when his proposals were opposed in Cabinet and several newspapers were calling for his resignation, Attlee gave Bevan his unwavering support both in and out of cabinet. Dalton as Chancellor of the Exchequer had to find the funds to finance the NHS. This he did "with a song in my heart". Dalton was wholly supportive of Bevan's vision of the NHS. If Bevan was the architect of the NHS, Dalton can be considered its midwife. The other essential figure in the formation of the NHS is John Maynard Keynes. Following President Truman's sudden and unannounced cessation of Lend Lease, which had sustained the country during the war, Keynes negotiated a loan of $3.75 bn, without which it is unlikely the radical agenda of the 1945 government, including the NHS, could have been achieved.

But the vision and the achievement of founding the NHS was primarily Bevan's. In Peter Hennessey's words: "The fifth of July was one of <u>the</u> great days in British history... it was a day that transformed like no other before or since the lives and chances of the British people. Fifth July, 1948 was the second of Britain's finest hours in the brave and high-minded 1940s. Like the Battle of Britain, it was a statement of intent, a symbol of hope in a formidable self-confident nation."

References

Aneurin Bevan: *In Place of Fear*, 1952 Heinemann, pp 75 and 77.

The Life and Labour of the People in London. Ed Charles Booth, 1889-1903.

Jose Harris: *William Beveridge, A Biography.* OUP, 1977.

Peter Hennessy: *Never Again Britain 1945-1952*, Jonathan Cape 1992, p 143.

A National Health Service. Cmd 6502, HMSO 1944.

Royal Commission on the Poor Laws and Relief of Distresses. *Minority Report*, HMSO 1909.

Seebohm Rowntree: *Poverty: A Study of Town Life*, 1901.

Arnold White: *Efficiency and Empire*, 1901, p102-103.

4

A prudent social model of health and care

Professor Sir Mansel Aylward CB

Sir Mansel is the Chair of the Bevan Commission and Chair of the Life Sciences Hub Wales. He is Director of the Centre for Psychosocial and Disability Research at Cardiff University and Professor for Prudent Health and Well-being at Swansea University. He was previously Chair of Public Health Wales – a unified NHS Trust responsible for the delivery of public health services at national, local and community level in Wales.

The case for change

The case for a different way of thinking and working and a more prudent model of health and wellbeing have been well rehearsed in part 1 of the Bevan Commissions *Exploiting the Legacy* series - *A New Way of Thinking* (Bevan Commission, 2017). This sets out why the more traditional models of service delivery do not help to alleviate the root causes and the underlying problems of many current day health and care issues.

With the challenges and threats to the future sustainability of health and health services in Wales and elsewhere, the notion of prevention and to some extent early intervention is a recurring theme in policy documents. Enabling individuals to lead healthier and more resilient lives is a clear and accepted goal as is promoting wellbeing rather than just treating ill health. However, the balance of resource and effort to date to reflect this goal is questionable. Similarly, the prominence of wellbeing rather than health reflects the move to focus on the individual rather than an individual's health problem.

The advent of the concept of Prudent Health Care (Bevan Commission, 2015) came at a time when on both the national and international stage a number of ideas, design principles and value based ways of working have been advanced and progressed to meet the need for robust, meaningful and workable models and initiatives to tackle more effectively the current demands on national health systems and to address the now well-articulated future burdens that frustrate the sustainability of these health services. The concept and principles of Prudent Health Care, or indeed a general prudent approach beyond the health care systems, does not conflict with the general thrust of this pursuit. Rather, the prudent approach provides an overarching basket in which each of these fit and enhance the proper application of the prudent model.

My fellow Bevan Commissioners and I believe this demands a social model based on the prudent principles in which everyone has a responsibility for health and must reflect and strongly address the determinants of ill health and the many other different factors which frustrate the attainment of people's maximum health and wellbeing.

The desired goal of healthcare is to eliminate or at the very least minimise the impacts of ill health and disabilities through effective and timely treatment and to enhance optimum functional recovery, as prudently as possible. It is about enabling people to do as much as possible as measured by functionality. The "achievement of health and wellbeing with the public, patients and professionals as equal partners through co-production" is an overarching basic tenet to be applied alongside the other three Prudent Health Care principles (Bevan Commission, 2015). This cannot be achieved within the confines of a strictly biomedical model which fails to include unique human attributes and the socio-economic determinants of ill health.

The most powerful determinants of (ill) health are social gradients (Marmot, 2004) and the linked problem of regional deprivation (Aylward and Phillips, 2008). My fellow Bevan Commissioner Professor Sir Michael Marmot will explore these later in this book. The prominence of wellbeing rather than health reflects the move to focus on the individual rather than an individual's health problem. This demands a social model which must reflect and strongly address the determinants of ill health and the many other different factors which frustrate the achievement of the people's wellbeing.

Conventional healthcare is, of course, important, but healthcare alone is not paramount in achieving good health and wellbeing. We have to recognise that improving health and wellbeing is not solely the responsibility of the NHS, but also should involve everyone. Our new way of thinking promotes the development of a health model which places responsibility for gaining good health beyond the NHS treatment service.

The move towards more person-centred care per se has become the favoured mantra of politicians and senior policy-makers in health for 20 years or longer. Person-centred care is not just about giving people whatever they want or just providing information. It is a way of thinking and doing things that sees the people using health and social services as equal partners in planning, developing and monitoring care to make sure it meets their needs. The Bevan

Commission believes that this still focuses upon doing things to people and for people and not with people, as promoted within the prudent health principles.

We seek to develop a health and care model which engenders a culture of ownership by all parties in decision-making and in gaining mutually agreed goals – an important characteristic of co-production and a key prudent health principle. It can promote health literacy and provide a framework for better clinical assessment, joint management of health, social and domestic matters, empowerment and enablement.

We must not hang onto the old ways of thinking and working; neither must we look for new and attractive answers that ignore the basic principles of Prudent Health and Care. We must be bold and take a different lens, a prudent lens, to find a model and approach that best suits the needs of people, preventing ill health, preserving and supporting wellbeing and providing a society that supports and enables us all to achieve these.

Conceptual models of health, illness and disability

Conceptual models of health, illness and disability are a practical approach to moving from theory to reality and a means of aiding understanding, management and research about what is required to deliver prudent health and healthcare for the people in Wales. These models help crystallise thinking, improve understanding and recognise the impact of human, social, environmental and economic implications. They can help develop joint decision making, facilitate co-production of solutions and engineer new interventions. Importantly they play a critical role in clarifying and formulating desired tangible outcomes and a sound framework for effective measurement and evaluation (Waddell and Aylward, 2010). Inevitably each model has its own strengths and weaknesses.

The current predominant biomedical model still provides the basis for our current healthcare system, reflecting the medicalisation of our population ("I have a health problem and need to see a doctor or other health professional who will make me better"), reinforcing this medicalisation of the health service, ("we have all these patients waiting for procedures, and I am measured on waiting times and throughput") and the medicalisation of our policy makers ("having more doctors and nurses would sort out the problems in the NHS").

The desired goal of healthcare is to eliminate or minimise the impacts of ill health and disabilities through effective and timely treatment and to enhance optimum functional recovery, as prudently as possible. The 'achievement of health and wellbeing with the public, patients and professionals as equal partners through co-production' is an overarching basic tenet to be applied alongside the other three prudent principles. This cannot be achieved within the confines of a strictly biomedical model which fails to include unique human attributes and the socio-economic determinants of ill health.

Social models and the role of personal and psychological factors provide a better understanding of health, wellbeing, sickness and disability. They also impact upon broader complex issues such as social exclusion, deprivation, capacity for work and developing interventions aimed at facilitating return to optimal health and the achievement of wellbeing. A social model of human illness that takes account of the person, their health problems and their social context has profound implications for healthcare, and social policy.

A bio-psychosocial model acknowledges that people may have a condition affecting their health, but the extent to which the health condition affects their ability to cope is affected by their wider social circumstances e.g. employment, education and skills, housing, relationships, environment and lifestyle, as well access to effective rehabilitation following illness. If we are to maximise the wellbeing and functioning of the population, then it is essential that we must ensure that the activities of all aspects of public life and the public sector which serves them are equally important.

The close links between social exclusion, disadvantage and poverty and the challenges faced by people with disabilities and illnesses frequently do not lie solely within the confines of the attributed diagnosed health condition. The impact on the individual person brought by the social and economic circumstances and the way society and the healthcare system are organised and delivered cannot be ignored. Conventional healthcare is, of course, important but healthcare alone is not paramount in achieving good health and wellbeing.

Medical versus social model

'Medicine has to some extent become a victim of its own 'life-saving' success and as a result it presents us with uncomfortable moral and ethical dilemmas', (Elliot, 2011). It drives a medical model of care which places the 'power' with the professionals delivering care rather than the individual receiving it. Blaming health professionals for this, while fashionable, is inappropriate.

The health service is sometimes wrongly perceived and often misunderstood by the population at large, as well as by politicians, as the primary actor with responsibility for improving health. Moreover, it is questionable and increasingly acknowledged by general practitioners that when dealing with the medical complaints are given insufficient time to explore fully a person's holistic health and social problems in a 7-10 minute consultation. The health service is regularly criticised for not doing enough to promote care in the community to reduce unnecessary admissions to hospital with the inevitable excessive demands on hospital care. Equally, this desired shift will bring demands on the services provided by local authorities where currently the patient's passage across such boundaries is fraught with difficulties when the needs of the patient may be lost in the process.

A social model perspective provides a different viewpoint and way of looking at and understanding health and care needs. It embeds a holistic approach on how we view people as individuals with a wide range of different needs and circumstances. It is complex and multi-faceted and does not lend itself to being discretely identified but presents as bundles of complex health and social care provided by a range of different agencies (local government, NHS and the third sector) and often changing over time.

A social model will take account of these wider barriers and obstacles and enable individuals to achieve their maximum potential physically, mentally and socially. A social model emphasises societal responsibility, exploits the social conscience which we cherish in Wales: focusing on each individual's circumstances and needs, but ensuring that all of the public sector, the third sector and indeed the private sector, are all committed to a common purpose through a prudent approach to health and wellbeing which necessarily does not neglect the importance brought by social care, rehabilitation, self-care, carer support, employment, education and skills, leisure services and housing.

The development and execution of this prudent social model requires robust joined up thinking across policy, organisational and professional boundaries to maximise the potential of the individual, their health, their locus of control and their economic success.

Legacy barriers to change

We have seen a continued failure by government to join up health, social care, employment, housing, welfare and education. This, combined with ingrained professional attitudes are powerful barriers to achieving the approaches seen in a social model, as are the views of the public, who can be equally inhibiting and at times irrational. In theory, when asked, the public may want to have more say over services, but in practice few actually get involved. It is often only in a crisis situation that mobilises large scale public involvement, which can result in corresponding political action. The challenge therefore remains as to how we ensure that that we effectively rebalance the relationship between the citizens and the state in a meaningful and prudent way.

When things go spectacularly and publicly wrong, as they did in the cases of GP Harold Shipman or the Mid Staffordshire NHS Foundation Trust, the instinctive policy and political response, for understandable reasons, has been primarily to enhance safety and protection through increased regulation, rather than to liberate and empower.

Additionally, finance will always be an important consideration and we all have a responsibility to ensure that we get the very best we can from the total resources available to us. Spending public resources wisely, prioritised according to greatest need is difficult, especially when we also have to consider the balance between prevention, early intervention, treatment and care, from the young to the elderly. While there is inevitably an emphasis on finance and financial regimens, this differs between macro level in health and the micro individual budgets seen within Social Care. These are driven by the different ways in which these sectors of care are financed, organised and delivered.

While more 'joined up' and integrated working is also often highlighted in policy, and indeed by the Commission, the disparity in the way different elements of care are financed and delivered are major barriers that must be overcome to ensure care is based upon the individual's health and social care needs and is fair and sustainable for everyone, irrespective of their position in society.

What we need is a better-balanced combination of all models; one simple and clear model which sets out what is required and how everyone can contribute, redrawing the relationship between the citizen and the state and rebalancing rights and responsibilities.

A common purpose and vision for Wales – A prudent model of health and wellbeing

People live their lives within wider family, community and work contexts. They are influenced by the people they come into contact with: their family, friends and workmates and through the wider environments that they are exposed to as they grow from children to adults through schools, universities and into society and the workplace.

The Bevan Commission have set out its thinking of what a Prudent Model of Health and Care should look like (Figure 1) This Welsh model of health and care is designed around the needs of people in Wales not the systems the processes or the professionals. It embraces the principles set out by Aneurin

Bevan for a National Health Service, namely; comprehensive, free at the point of delivery and accessible by all, alongside the fundamental 4 Prudent Principles.

This prudent model of health and social care will:

- actively encourage everyone to take collective action and responsibility to help us all live the healthiest lives for as long as possible;
- call upon all agencies to act together and assume joint responsibility in whatever way they can best do this to ensure we make the most of the resources we have to meet individual and population health needs;
- develop a strong, robust and prudent integrated health and care system to support both our health and care needs;
- ensure that we make the most effective use of all skills and resources available including local people, patients and the third sector; and
- ensure that those with greatest needs are prioritised and to ensure that there are no, so called, 'hard to reach' groups in society.

A prudent health and care system is one in which we all share responsibility for maintaining our health and that of others and that we have a high quality, effective and efficient service which meets the needs of people, as and when needed.

Figure 1 – A prudent cooperative health and care system for Wales
(Bevan Commission, 2018)

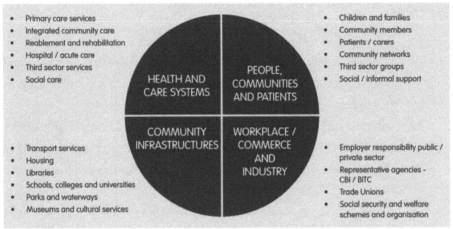

In summary

Engaging with and gaining the support of all partners in this shared vision will be crucial to its success. A prudent model of health and health care will need widespread sign up and active support from the public sector, private industry, life sciences, the third sector and the public itself if we are to achieve better health and wellbeing for people in Wales. The transformation and integration of thinking, service design and service delivery must also form key features of a future model that should find places for, and strongly encourage and facilitate ongoing innovation, research and learning, where evaluation of effectiveness using data and public/patient outcomes are intrinsic to collaborative working.

Postscript

The chapter draws from the first two papers in the Bevan Commission's Heritage series and was largely drafted before the final report of the Parliamentary Review into Health and Care in Wales was published.

However, it provides a clear and detailed response to the Review's call for the development of new models of health and care.

References

Aylward M. & Phillips C.J. (2008). *Report for Edwina Hart AM MBE, Minister for Health and Social Services*. Welsh Assembly Government.

Bevan Commission (2015) Prudent Health Principles.

Bevan Commission (2017). *A New Way of Thinking: The Need for a Prudent Model for Health and Care*.

Bevan Commission (2018). *A New Way of Planning: Working towards a Prudent Model for Health and Care*.

Elliot J. (2011). *Moving beyond the medical model Journal of holistic healthcare*. Available at: http://www.martinsey.org.uk/pdf/moving.pdf.

Marmot M. (2004). *Status Syndrome*. London: Bloomsbury.

5

Prudent health and social care – people and their needs

Nygaire Bevan

Nygaire is the great niece of Aneurin Bevan, the creator of the NHS, and was named after him. After qualifying as nurse her career led her to working with people with learning disabilities, older people, children with disabilities and troubled young people. She was previously Assistant Director for Powys County Council and with Powys Local Health Board as a Locality Manager. She currently is a board member for the Care Council for Wales and has worked with the Social Services Improvement Agency which forms part of the WLGA.

I have been asked to complete this chapter for this anniversary book of the NHS for its 70th birthday and I have been doing a little thinking – what would our world be like without the NHS? What would Nye think of it all now?

So, some key questions to pose: Where would we go to see a GP, what type of service would it be – online, skype contact? Would we see the same one or a different one every time? How would we pay for the drugs they prescribe and how much would they cost? Would there be a community nurse to support your vulnerable mother at home?

What would happen if a member of your family had a heart attack? Would there be ambulances staffed with qualified paramedics or would you be expected to bundle your loved one in the car (if you have one) and get them to the nearest (may be miles away) hospital which may or may not have the expert facilities to treat your relative. And throughout this episode, you may have to produce evidence of how you would pay before treatment starts, are worried and concerned as well as the dreaded fear of how much you will need to pay and how you will pay it. Will I need to take out a loan, will I get into debt?

How would we have managed at the Manchester bombing or the London Bridge terror attack without the blue light services and those professionals who went above and beyond their duties to save lives and bring order back to our cities? My hunch is many more would have died and those cities would have been in chaos.

We must also remember the significant contribution of the entire professional, office and all other staff who are part of the NHS and what contribution they make to the tax and national insurance receipts. These staff will also impact the economies of their local communities and country by spending, saving and buying products. Then there are the army of people who are employed to build our MRI scanners, pack the syringes, build our ambulances and feed our patients, whose contribution to the GDP must be huge.

As you would expect I am a strong advocate of the NHS and I believe it is the best in the world. However, it does have its challenges as we have seen daily over this Winter period, as we do each year. We are all aware of the pressures of this political hot potato – increasing demand, people living longer with a range of complex needs, rising expectations of the public, new technology and medical advances etc., and we really need to have a serious conversation with the public about what the NHS will and will not do.

If one were to ask a few people in the street where they would want to be if they were ill, most would say in their own homes, cared for by those they love. Now that's fine if you have the flu but if you have a brain tumour you will need specialist diagnosis, specialist surgery and maybe specialist aftercare treatment in the form of radiotherapy and chemotherapy. The same could be said if it were a stroke, specialist diagnosis, intensive physiotherapy and drug treatments. My point here is that acute care is normally a very small proportion of people's experience with the NHS and they return to live at home as soon as they can – it is primary and social care that is there 'for the long haul' and community support and resilience needs to be the focus. We cannot continue putting millions and millions into secondary care and doing the 'same old', while the situation continues to get worst and nothing changes.

Social care meets the needs of a range of people and issues from the most simple to the most complex. It provides information and advice at the front door to enable people to be more empowered to make their own decisions. It also carries out complex assessment – for example mental capacity and Deprivation of Liberty Safeguards (DoLS).

Following assessment, social care also provides and funds a range of services to allow people to remain living at home (domiciliary care), supports them to get better and improve (re-ablement) and identifies the right environment if people need to enter residential or nursing care. It supports all client groups from the very young to the very old, with varying needs and aspirations. As part of the local authority family, social care is best placed to access those other services, housing, sport and leisure, to holistically support the wellbeing of the individual. However, there is duplication in this service which, if managed better, could provide a better service to individuals and potentially be more efficient.

It was against this backdrop that the Bevan Commission spent time developing the prudent principles. As the principals seek a system-wide approach and recognises inter-dependence is it very pertinent to this chapter on health and social care integration.

Figure 1 – A prudent cooperative health and care system for Wales
(Bevan Commission, 2018)

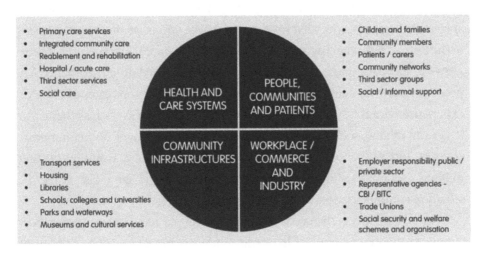

Illness is neither an indulgence for which people have to pay, nor an offence for which they should be penalised, but a misfortune, the cost of which should be shared by the community.

Aneurin Bevan

Integrating health and social care for the future

So, what's the solution? I am now in the fortunate position of being retired and having worked in social care and health all my working life I can safely say, (and without repercussions), "It ain't working." I can list pages of policies, legislative change, strategies – Community Care Act, Social Services and Wellbeing (Wales) Act, National Service Frameworks (for every condition – strokes, diabetes, mental health etc. with targets and demands), Fulfilled Lives, Supportive Communities, *Beecham Report*, Future Generations Act Wales and the latest the Parliamentary Review of Health and Social Care – and there are many, many more. No sooner are you implementing one that another tranche hits the desk. So, one of the big messages for me in this chapter is a plea to politicians that producing a shiny new policy does not mean that things will improve – in fact things may get worse.

So, to get back to the question – how do we integrate health and social care? We have created a difficult landscape for future change which will require brave and courageous leaders who have permissions and freedoms to act. Governance, budgets, free at the point of delivery / charging, continuing health care, terms and conditions of staff and many other blocks must be overcome. The public are not concerned with many of these issues (paying for care may be the only concern for them), what they want is the best for their loved ones.

BUT... it can work. I have personal experience of losing a husband and both parents to major disease, cancer and stroke. They all chose to be cared for and die at home and their wishes were granted. So, what made this work in a very rural area of Wales which it could be said would be more of a challenge? It worked because there was joined up health and social care with the local GPs taking the lead. The necessary equipment arrived, district nurse and occupational therapist supported, social workers organised the care package, palliative care support was available when required and everyone communicated with each other. Professional preciousness was not apparent, the family's needs were at the centre and those most poorly paid of all, the domiciliary carers, provided the highest care and treated my family members with dignity and respect.

The integration of health and social care is not new and it has developed in areas of Wales and England. In Wales, many health boards are planning for this change. Local authorities have taken a significant reduction in budgets over many years. This required a root and branch analysis of what services were statutory so legally have to be provided, identification of areas where there were opportunities to reduce services or charge more for them and they organised a programme to consult with the public and the workforce. This required some brave decision-making for leaders who needed to 'cut their cloth' to the money distributed from Welsh Government.

The report by Wales Public Services highlights that per capita spending on social care has fallen in real terms by 13% over the last five years in Wales. Spending per head would have to increase by at least £134 million (24%) between 2015-16 and 2020-21 to return to the equivalent level of spending in 2009-10, which amounts to a 3.7% year-on-year increase.

The issue for the NHS is that many of the Local Health Boards are not coming in on budget so additional significant money continues to be given to it each year. To me they are failing to demonstrate how they will reduce the waste and duplication in the NHS system and are not even able to identify one or two areas that they will analyse in depth to make any the changes necessary. And there are lots of opportunities – estates, prescribing, transport, and use of agency staff to name a few. The service seems to be in constant crisis mode and although they will have strategic plans in place they are often undelivered because of operational demands. Leadership, capacity, skill level and a freedom to act independently from central government (national health) control may also be a big challenge for LHBs.

What and where next

The NHS touches everyone, from childbirth, treating disease and long term conditions. It treats the very young to the very old and in most cases, considering the numbers of people that access it on a daily basis; it does a pretty good job. The NHS treats the most not the few.

However, there are still factors and pressures that are holding us back:

- We need to work faster and sharper and work in a more whole systems approach (realising that we all have a key role in service delivery for vulnerable people along with others). We cannot do it alone;
- Our focus needs to be on sustainable service improvement;
- There needs to be political and leadership drive to make things happen quicker;
- Serious financial pressures for all the partners' means we need to work together if we are to achieve the change we need. We at least need to test it out to prove it will or will not work;
- Transitional, long term funding is needed to allow us to modernise services at community levels in a whole systems way as required by the major policies;
- Inspection and regulation should complement and support local authorities and health boards while they undertake this change, as well as being a quality check for the public.

I have experience, as many of us do, of being a patient of the NHS at both primary and secondary care levels. I have also throughout my career worked alongside health professionals in my social care practitioner and management roles. There is a lot we can do to make it better and I do think that we now taking liberties and advantage of this very special service. I am not saying anything new here, it has all been said before, I am just frustrated that we can't seem to do something about it.

I would fully support integration; it should avoid duplication and improve efficiencies. It won't, however, save huge amounts of money but it will improve the service and quality for the individual.

Coming back to Nye, I think he would say the NHS has been a service of significant impact at an individual, community, national and international level. It has saved lives and kept people well for longer. What it now needs is a complete relook and a total rethink on what it needs to look like for this, and future generations. We need to loosen the straitjacket of politics and politicians need to support the case for change at local levels. Leaders need to lead, boards need hold leaders to account, and we need to get on with it. We have all the evidence that we need for change. Finally, we need to have a true and realistic debate with the public.

6

Maintaining health and wellbeing in communities

Professor Kamila Hawthorne
MBE MD FRCGP FRCP FAcadMEd DRCOG DCH

Kamila is a GP, Associate Dean for Medicine at the University of Surrey, and Vice Chair (Professional Development) at the Royal College of General Practitioners. Her research interests and publications include access to health services for Black and Minority Ethnic and other disadvantaged groups in the UK (with special application to Type 2 Diabetes), the development of social responsibility in health care professionals, and equality and diversity in medical education assessments.

The people of Wales live in communities, and their individual health and wellbeing is clearly linked to the health and wellbeing of their neighbourhoods (Barton and Grant, 2006). A growing elderly population, enduring inequalities in health, increasing numbers of patients with complex chronic and multiple conditions, rising obesity rates and a challenging financial climate pose some real threats and challenges to maintaining our sustainability and good health to create a prosperous, successful Wales.

While primary care provides the interface between the community and health and social care, secondary care provides specialist services for patients with illness and/or disability. As the diagram below shows (Figure 1),

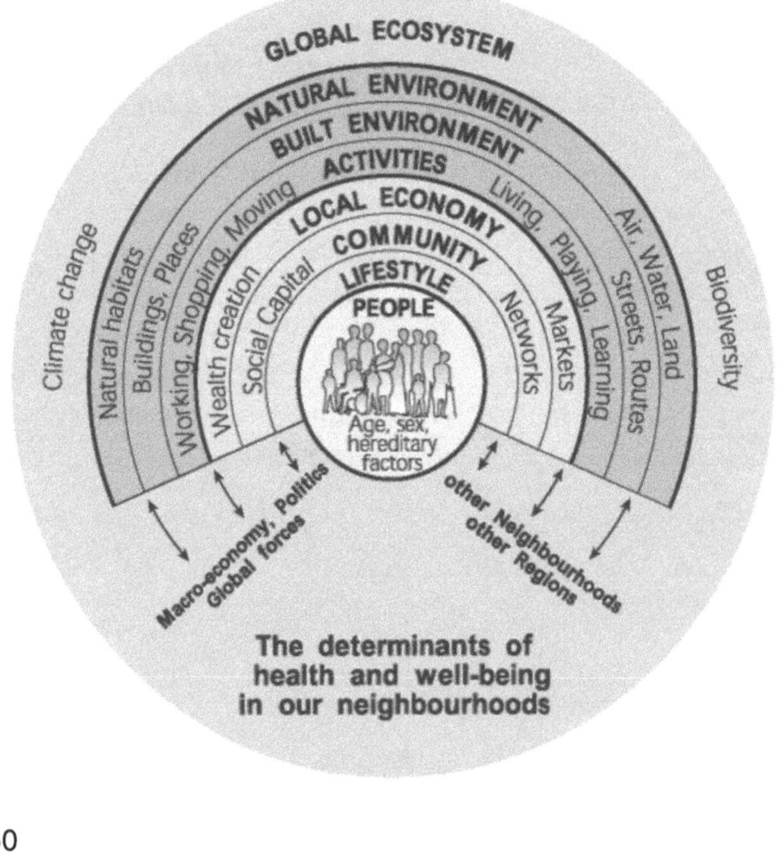

Figure 1 - The determinants of health and wellbeing in our neighbourhoods

healthcare systems only directly feed into the core (the four inner sections) concentric circles of determinants of health.

Barbara Starfield (2005) demonstrated the cost effectiveness of national healthcare systems that are primary-care led, and identified its key features as being the first point of contact for most health problems, co-ordination of care for individuals, but particularly that it provides holistic, comprehensive longitudinal care delivered in the context of family and community. While community services are delivered by a multiplex of organisations, both statutory and voluntary, the 'essence' of a community comes from its members alone and their willingness to behave as a social, cohesive and supportive unit.

Research from Wales *(Caerphilly Health and Social Needs Study)* has shown that living in deprived neighbourhoods, where there is poor quality housing, poor access to amenities, and where neighbourhood safety and behaviour is an issue, all affect measures of self-reported physical and mental health. The Welsh Assembly Government funded 'Communities First' project (WAG, 2001), was a programme of neighbourhood regeneration in the 100 most deprived electoral wards in Wales, that recognised the importance of building and retaining strong, cohesive communities in the health of individuals and shows that strategies to improve health of communities should be targeted as much at 'place' as at 'people'.

The Welsh Assembly must promote and protect positive health in a much more personalised way, working in co-production with specified communities across Wales. The NHS needs to re-design itself to become much more engaged in the wider agenda outlined here, working outside its historical and traditional 'biomedical model' to bring in a much more holistic and socially responsive service that follows a more prudent social model of health as advocated by the Bevan Commission. A key element would be a workforce trained to think differently, to problem-solve and to be prepared to work with patients and the public to ensure that the differing needs of different communities are met. The same applies to Local Government, the Third Sector and other agencies, and the people of Wales, themselves. But it needs to be led by the Welsh Government. 'Together for Health' (WG, 2011) invited the people of Wales to join with the Welsh Assembly to create a Wales where health matches the best anywhere – but, without leadership, this remains a vision and not a reality.

Services that best serve people's health and wellbeing needs

A few key principles need to be considered in developing and delivering a service that is best suited to the needs of the population:

- We know that the public wishes their health care to be delivered at or near to their homes and communities.
- We need to target services to those who are most needy, as well as delivering comprehensive coverage to all. Careful management of this strategy is needed to ensure it remains effective, and can flex with changes in demography and need of the population. In particular:
  - Within 15 years, one in three people in Wales will be aged over 60 years, and the number of older frail people over 75 will have increased by 76%. As people age, they develop chronic conditions, multi-morbidity and increasingly complex management needs, both medical and social.
  - Maternal and child health services remain vital to support young families and give them the start in life they need to remain healthy.
  - Learning difficulties/ mental health also continues to be a significant aspect of health needs, often hidden from view, and often not resourced adequately.
- Life expectancy for the most deprived 1/5th of the population has risen more slowly than for any other group – for example, there remains a 10-year difference in average lifespan for people in

Cyncoed and Butetown; both areas of the same city, Cardiff. Public health initiatives to help tackle obesity at all ages, smoking, drinking and substance misuse are much needed, as well as clear and well publicised health promotion strategies in which statutory bodies work with the public to change behavioural norms. We know this can be done, as evidenced by the fall in teenage pregnancy rates in Wales, the change in attitudes to smoking in public places and to drinking and driving.

- Combining health and social care such that the boundaries cease to be recognised.
- Health and social care are increasingly being recognised as facets of the same, holistic service. One cannot exist without the other, and deficiencies in one can seriously affect the working of the other.
- This has been evidenced by the build-up of ambulances waiting at A&E doorways, due to bed shortages in hospitals as consultants are employed on 'discharge' ward rounds, to move patients who no longer need hospital-based care but are too frail or sick to manage at home. Lengthy delays in discharging patients due to problems with resourcing social care are a clear indication of the relationship between health and social care. Conversely, without a community-based healthcare workforce (for example, District Nurses, Community Dieticians and Physiotherapists, Community Mental Health Nurses), many patients who receive help with social care (carers who come in several times a day to feed, wash and monitor frail patients at home), would not be able to manage.
- Medical and healthcare education in general needs to move with the times. It is still too biomedical in its approach and a holistic consulting model is much spoken of, but not practised sufficiently. Medical students need to be shown role models working in community settings who can enthuse them to see the benefits and

job satisfaction that can come from day to day encounters with patients in communities other than examples from heroic surgery or complex interventions with new and expensive drugs. A new generation of healthcare workers who are able to work in co-production with patients and the public, who 'think outside the box' when it comes to a medical presentation that might have social undertones such as domestic violence, poor social support, loneliness and isolation, and have the tools to hand to offer help that is more than a temporary 'sticking plaster' that will otherwise result in the patient bouncing back days, weeks or months later.

- Resource allocation should follow strategic planning. If the aim is to keep people out of expensive secondary care beds, then resources should be targeted at health promotion to prevent illness and maintain health and wellbeing, early diagnosis of illness and new models of care that allow patients to be cared for either at home by specially trained multi-disciplinary teams, in local community hospitals or in 'step-down' wards if they need rehabilitation prior to discharge.

- The management of health and social services also needs careful review, and streamlining to reduce bureaucracy, strengthen integration and enable quick and effective decision-making. Management needs to be able to grasp what opportunities there are, to shape and improve services.

Making the most of all skills and resources

The practice of health and social care in the future will involve 'connected health'; using digital and communications technology to deliver cost-effective solutions at a time when the demands on health and social care services continue to increase. This applies to community settings as much as to secondary care. Digital health, including wearables, monitors and apps, has the capacity to provide new models of care, that use artificial intelligence and Big Data to monitor patients with chronic conditions from home, and to use risk-analysis algorithms to predict events before they happen, and prevent them.

Patients are the single most important users of health apps currently, and 75% of the UK population goes on line for health information, mostly looking for information on symptoms and medical conditions. Responding to this need with trustworthy, accurate data, easy to use technology and guarantee of data security, could give health providers a lever to co-produce health with patients and needs to be exploited. IT solutions can minimise paperwork and save time for hard pressed doctors and nurses, increase patient face-time and reduce unnecessary hospital admissions. In addition to minimizing avoidable service use, it improves outcomes, promotes patient independence and can focus on prevention.

NHS England, the RCGP and the Kings Fund have all supported the role of general practitioners (GPs) both in dealing with additional demand for services in primary care, and in taking a more proactive role in ill-health prevention and public health. There are national imperatives to push for increases in GPs entering the profession as well as for new ways to retain GPs who would otherwise retire early. In all four countries, the NHS is moving to substantially increase the numbers of paramedics, nurses, community pharmacists, physiotherapists and physician associates in the primary care skill-mix. This can help free up GPs to deal with more complex medical cases and give them headspace to express their potential in leading multi-disciplinary teams to deliver new models of working, and the strategic aims for Primary and Community Care in Wales.

The recent Inquiry into Primary Care Clusters in Wales (Health, Social Care and Sport Committee, National Assembly for Wales, Oct 2017) has identified some impressive examples of work in specific clusters across Wales, but concludes "that systemic change in the way primary care meets local needs is still needed, and that clusters have a long way to go before they can play a significant role in planning the transfer of services and resources out of hospitals and into local communities." These include facilitating the creation of federations of practices with integrated skill-mix health and social care teams, and community care hubs. Effective and flexible health and social care partnerships that can deliver some of the social prescribing / engineering activities related to housing, training, employment and social cohesion activities described earlier in this section, are urgently needed and should be supported.

Overall, investment in general practice has fallen to about 8% of the NHS Wales budget, somewhat short of the 11% that was available to general practice 10 or more years ago. Over this time, investment in specialist care has increased, while numbers of GPs have fallen. It has become imperative to attract, recruit and retain GPs, to match population demand due changing demography, rises in unscheduled care and shifting care into the community. There are few or no applicants for what were previously competitive posts in primary care. Many practices across Wales have to make do with expensive and inadequate locum services (a GP locum cannot provide the same service as a GP principal), sacrificing the precious values of general practice, such as continuity of care and easy access. Investment in GP premises has fallen and many premises owned by GP principals are barely fit for purpose for today's healthcare needs, let alone tomorrow's demands. Removal of GP 24-hour responsibility in 2004, and poor funding decisions, has resulted in a largely privatised out-of-hours service that is chronically understaffed and overstretched.

Re-orientation and refocusing of NHS Wales' resources is needed, if the financial envelope really cannot be stretched any further. More GPs with time and skills to lead change and innovation in primary care have to be found, if the National Assembly for Wales' vision for a world-class healthcare service, delivered in or near patients' homes, is to be realised. The problem is now, and the problem is urgent.

References

Barton, H. & Grant, M. (2006). *A health map for the local human habitat. Journal of the Royal Society for the Promotion of Health*. 126(6): 252-253.

Health, Social Care and Sport Committee (2017) *Inquiry into Primary Care: Clusters*. National Assembly for Wales.

Starfield, B. (2005) *Contribution of Primary Care to Health Systems and Health*. Milbank Q. 2005 Sep; 83(3): 457–502.

Welsh Government (2011). Together for Health.

Welsh Assembly Government (2001). 'Communities First' Programme.

7

From hospital to home: Back to the future

Professor Dame Sue Bailey OBE DBE

Dame Sue is Chair of the Children and Young People's Mental Health Coalition, Honorary Professor of Mental Health Policy at the University of Central Lancashire; Chair of the Academy of Medical Royal Colleges; Senior Clinical Advisor for Mental Health at Health Education England; External Advisor to the Minister of Health and Social Care for the Review of CAMHS in Wales. Until recently, she was a Consultant Child and Adolescent Forensic Psychiatrist at Greater Manchester West NHS Foundation Trust. She was President of the Royal College of Psychiatrists from 2011 to 2014. During her time as President she worked with health and social care professionals, patients and carers to bring about Parity of Esteem between mental and physical health.

A personal view

The best chance of delivering a sustainable, place-based health and social care system is to think forward from now to the world of 2048. To do this, we need to apply the theory of change and create headspace to think beyond the day-to-day toil of performance targets and crises erupting across the system.

Whether it's the inevitability of a season called winter, pressures in primary care or simply the lived experience of human beings, there are always challenges facing a patient's journey through the meandering corridors of our hospitals. I believe that patients, carers and healthcare staff have a shared hope for the ability to live life well whatever the illness.

But the world beyond health and social care must understand that good community healthcare depends on there being decent housing and transport systems, supporting patients to live beyond their diagnoses and to have a sense of positive social connectedness.

What follows is my perspective on how we can achieve sustainable health care by working together.

The golden threads

A move from hospital to home will require, first and foremost, a move from organisational to cross-systems leadership. It will require understanding and acting upon not just the evidence base stemming from randomised control trials of single specific diseases, but also the knowledge we have accrued in real world medical practice. This will address the reality of the fast growth of the number of patients across the world living with multiple illnesses (MacMahon, 2018).

We must be bold about what this will mean for future education, training and support of the whole health and social care workforce. We need to emphasise the part that every child and citizen, in every family, in every street, across the UK can play in improving healthcare outcomes for themselves and the communities in which they live.

This requires a true mind-set change. All health and care professionals, policy makers and members of the public need to understand the benefits and embrace the critical importance of shared decision-making. We must not ask what can the medical science of the future offer us, but what should it be doing that is values-based and represents value for money.

To do this, we need to move beyond diagnosis but understand the impact of diseases on the functioning of the individual across all aspects of their life in their unique social circumstances.

We should all have the right to be more than our illnesses.

This requires a shift towards a social identity approach (Haslam, 2018) to healthcare that moves beyond the increasingly tired debate of whether health is a product of genes, environment or chance. What lies at the heart of the health of individuals is the nature of the social connections that exist between them, and the sense of shared identity that these connections both produce and are produced by (Haslam, 2018).

A social identity approach lays down the foundations of a new way of thinking and learning about how, as practitioners across the spheres of health, social care and education, we can truly develop better "ways of seeing" health. This in turn provides a platform for us to work with others to promote better "ways of being" in the world for the patients and public we serve (Berger, 1972).

From the first spark of life and throughout our lives, our mental and physical health is profoundly affected by the places we live, the people with whom we interact and the communities to which we belong. Across the world, governments and policy makers are increasingly recognising the importance of social life for the health of all citizens and turning themselves to the dual task of understanding these processes better and then using that understanding to build healthier societies (Gardner, 2016), (Haslam, 2018).

How then should we be developing the systems' leaders of the future and what are the enablers we can bring in to support them? Since the 1960s, in an attempt to "solve the problem of the NHS" (amidst the ever-ongoing organisational restructuring of the NHS, increased regulation and legislative changes) there have been slowly evolving attempts to embed clinical leadership across multidisciplinary teams. Only more recently have we seen serious attempts to create distributive leadership at all levels, across the patients' pathway of care from hospital to home.

To support systems leaders, we have to establish agreement on what it is we are trying to achieve, framed in realistic optimism. Continuous improvement in care requires population health that is values-based, value for money and done in partnership with the public.

We need to develop better knowledge of improvement methods and how to put them into practice across whole systems. Improvement must be incorporated into appraisals for medical professions and properly measured in evaluation. Systems should be put in place that support learning at local and regional levels as well as on a national scale, emphasising the power of peer-to-peer learning. Above all, it is vital to develop leaders drawn from many different professional groups who can share best practice in how to achieve high quality care in partnership.

Enabling environments and shared values

During the time I held the role of President of the Royal College of Psychiatrists (2011-2014) and subsequently as Chair of the Academy of Medical Royal Colleges (2015-2017), I had a unique opportunity to pull together strands of psychological thinking to support effective systems leaders of the future (RCpsych OP88 2013) (Herman, 2014) (Bailey, 2017). I was passionate about the role of Enabling Environments, values-based practice and shared decision-making.

Enabling Environments can:

- Improve quality of care and therefore measurable patient outcomes (Haas, 2000).

- Promote the wellbeing of patients, optimising conditions for recovery (Robinson, 2004).
- Enhance workforce engagement (Rondeau and Wagar, 2012).
- Reduce staff sick leave (Powell, 2014).
- Support positive mood and enable more effective teamwork (Manser, 2009).
- Increase productivity (Department of Health, 2009).

The challenge is how then can Enabling Environments be delivered not just across an organisation but across a whole health and care system? The answer is: by utilising values based practice and shared decision-making.

As a developmental psychiatrist and social scientist, I approach what follows by referring to what we could do to deliver sustainable health for the next generation: the voters, parents, educationalists and health and social care workers of 2048.

Human rights and values-based practice should be at the heart of all health services and have been piloted in surgery and radiology. Autonomy, control and participation are all key, with human rights values protected by the right to respect private life.

In 2016, the Royal College of Psychiatrists, the Children and Young People's Mental Health Coalition (which I am privileged to chair) and Young Minds came together to take evidence from across the UK, as the Child and Adolescent Mental Health Systems Values-Based Commission. This grouping enabled us to develop a framework of shared values in partnership with those whose needs are being considered i.e. acting in the best interest of children and young people and meeting their mental health needs.

Another example of developing shared values is Choosing Wisely, a well-established international campaign that was kick-started in the UK as Prudent Healthcare in Wales and Realistic Medicine in Scotland. Choosing Wisely UK was developed by the Academy of Royal Medical Colleges, in collaboration with partners across all parts of the healthcare system, to enable better conversations between patients and their clinicians regarding tests, treatments and procedures. This initiative enabled the patient to choose care that is: supported by evidence, not duplicative of other tests and procedures, free from harm, truly necessary and consistent with their values.

When training medical students (who will work as generalists in the community in the future), we need to make a major shift in how they listen and learn from their patients who have the unique experience of their illness. Patients will hold their own attitudes towards risks when it comes to treatment options, aligned to their own goals and values. When they come to talk about prognosis they will want to know how their needs will be met in their treatment, in a way that respects them as individuals.

Supporting systems leadership through innovation and training

So, what is the offer on the table to improve systems leadership from research, innovation and new technology?

In the 70th year of the NHS we have a solid digital-first foundation driven by the internet, social media, mobile technologies and big data. Soon we can also add cognitive systems, nanotechnology and robotics to the list. How will these emerging technologies prove essential to the health and care system?

As 5G hospitals become a reality, we must also consider how next-generation digital technologies can improve operational flow and patient care beyond geographical boundaries. Soon we will be able to integrate task management systems, automate processes, connect services and track patients, assets and employees.

I believe that higher education institutions, in particular, have an important role to play in developing fit-for-purpose systems leaders who can meet these technological challenges and opportunities. Our educators need to be equipping the future workforce and upskilling the extant workforce to: concentrate and focus deeply; solve problems through cooperative networks;

search for information; discern the quality of information and to communicate findings effectively (Grogan, 2018).

Above all, educators of the future will need to equip individuals and teams to develop an adaptive mind-set, critical thinking and social intelligence, enabling them to connect with people and take initiative for their own learning.

We are at the start of an educational revolution where medicine cannot fall behind; therefore, we need a new technical and professional workforce. To deliver this revolution, the workforce needs the time and headspace to learn. Learning by 2025 will be based on competencies, capabilities, attitudes and intelligences - supported by disciplinary knowledge. But above all, our workforce must develop transferable skills, personal resilience, social and cultural capital and conscious curiosity.

Integrated health and social care

A major barrier to delivering systems leadership for the next generation is being able and willing to fund social care across the lifespan. For the immediate future, a conversation is needed that gives us the opportunity to explore and develop shared expectations across governments, professionals, public and patients of what social care can and or should deliver. It does, however, require an honest and informed discussion about funding at all ages and stages of life.

This is about more than the needs of frail elders, but about quality and safety embedded in practice and whole person integrated care. This would necessitate a well-supported provider network and a well-supported workforce capitalising on shared learning and practice across health and social care. It requires practical support for families and carers, including empowering them with evidence-based knowledge.

All potential solutions that necessitate funding are challenging, but we could start to explore how we could pool risk to address the unpredictable nature of care costs.

As we know, health inequalities do not arise by chance and cannot simply be attributed to genetic makeup, unhealthy behaviour or even barriers to accessing to health care. All of these factors are important, but overall it is the conditions of people's daily lives that shape their health behaviours and health outcomes. Unequal distribution of money, power and resources shape these conditions of daily life.

So how do we move beyond the polarised political debates? We could start with the needs of children and young people. What could make a real difference across child health is a non-stigmatising approach to support the improvement of parenting, which has to include at its core the improvement of parents' lives (Bush, 2018). Where better to start than to work in common cause across the whole of child health? The impact of inequality is seen in childhood across a range of both physical and mental health conditions (including obesity, oral health, cancer, mental health and birth weight), and therefore needs to be addressed holistically (Donkin, 2018) (Young Minds, 2018) (WHO, 2011).

A way forward

Whilst it is positive that there is currently a light being shone on mental health, we need to understand how it can act as a support to help health systems leadership for better overall healthcare outcomes.

The World Health Organisation defines good mental health as a state of wellbeing in which every individual realises his or her potential, copes with the normal stresses of life, works productively and fruitfully and is able to contribute to his or her own community.

While no one could argue with this statement in principle, we often diverge from it in our actions.

Are we brave enough as a society to really move the emphasis, the funding and the workforce from hospital to home? Or will we continue to acknowledge what we need to do but not act as we must?

The future of society relies on how we empower and support young people to be the adults of 2048, who see good mental health and wellbeing as a basic right, but also to enable them to do what will likely be expected of them. It is critical that the next generation of health and care professionals recognise the importance of moving care from hospital to the home, and possess the intelligent kindness needed to do it.

Ballat and Campling (2013) wrote about 'Intelligent Kindness' in part to respond to what many viewed as a negative event (the Health and Social Care Act of 2012), but they retained enough realistic optimism to describe how systems leaders could and should function to deliver improved health care outcomes.

In the same way, in *A Manifesto for a Healthy and Health Creating Society* (Crisp, 2016), which was published in the wake of Brexit, the authors laid out a positive vision for health and care in the UK to counterbalance prevailing pessimism. In writing about moving health and care from hospital to home, I hope I have touched on the four themes of their Manifesto paper:

- How the UK could and should strengthen its role as a global centre for health and biomedical life sciences.
- The transformation of the health and care system from a hospital-centred and illness-based system to a person-centred and health-based system.
- The development and implementation of a plan for building a health-creating society, supported by all sectors of the economy and wider population that addresses health inequalities.
- How health, care and scientific institutions should help restore a healthy society in the UK.

The New Psychology of Health: Unlocking the Social Cure (Haslam, 2018) has now almost 70 years of research and evidence sat behind it, but for the first time has applied the social identity approach to all parts of medicine.

With shared social identity and positive group behaviour, we can shift the focus to 'we and us' from the 'I and me' model. We can build social and psychological resources that can provide a sense of connection, purpose and control in our lives, whatever our illnesses, enabling us to achieve enhanced health and wellbeing.

If we lose social identity or develop a harmful, toxic social identity, our health and wellbeing will be compromised. Returning to the WHO definition of mental health and the much-welcomed attention being given to children and young people's mental health, we can agree that wellbeing brings with it the four essential components of a healthy progression through adolescence and into adulthood (Shooter, in Bailey, Tarbuck and Chitsabesan, 2017):

- A sense of control in your life;
- An ability to communicate;
- An ability to cooperate; and
- The ability to compromise.

We can only secure the long-term sustainability of the UK health and care system if we can grow systems leaders, at all levels and across all geographies, who understand and act to reduce morbidity, create a healthier population and help build resilient communities. To do this, they will need to develop shared values and goals with the communities in which they are working. I have every confidence that they will rise to meet that challenge with enthusiasm and kindness.

References

Bush, M. *Addressing Adversity: Prioritising adversity and trauma informed care for Children and Young People in England Young Minds - NHS Health*. Education. England (2018).

Bailey. *Looking Back to the Future the re-emergence of green care. BJPSYCH International* volume 14 number 4 -79, 2017.

Ballatt, J. and Campling, P. (2013). *Intelligent Kindness - Reforming the Culture of Healthcare*. Royal College of Psychiatrists publications.

Berger, J. *Ways of Seeing*. Penguin Classics, 1972, reprinted 2008.

Haas, J. S. *Is the Professional Satisfaction of General Internists Associated with Patient Satisfaction?* 2000.

Haslam, A. and Haslam, C. *The New Psychology of Health: Unlocking the Social Cure*. Routledge, 2018.

Herman H. (2014) *Editorial the central place of psychiatry in healthcare*. Acta Psychiatrica. Scandinavia. 129 401-403.

Department of Health. *Departmental Report*. 2009.

Donkin A. J. M. (in press) in Eds. Shaw M. and Bailey S. *Justice for children, a developmental perspective*. Chapter the Social Determinants of Health. Cambridge University Press.

Enabling Environments CCQI at the RCPsych.

Gardner, C. *Citizenship, Recovery and Inclusive Society Partnership (CRISP) to shed new light on social inclusion and health. Yale Programme for Recovery and Community Health,* Published 2016, (Accessed April 2018)

MacMahon, S. *Multimorbidity: a priority for global health research*. Academy of Medical Sciences, 2018.

Manser, T. *Teamwork and patient safety in dynamic domains of healthcare: a review of the literature*. 2009.

Robinson, D. G. *Symptomatic and functional recovery from a first episode of schizophrenia or schizoaffective disorder*. 2004.

Rondau, K. and Wagar, T. *Employee High-Involvement Work Practices and Voluntary Turnover: Does Human Capital Accumulation or an Employee Empowerment Culture Mediate the Process? Examining the Evidence in Canadian Healthcare Organizations*. 2012.

Royal College of Psychiatry OP88 (2013) *Whole-person care from Rhetoric to Reality, Achieving parity between mental and physical health*. Rcpsych publications.

Powell, M., Dawson, J., Topakas, A., Durose, J. and Fewtrell, C. *Staff satisfaction and organisational performance: evidence from a longitudinal secondary analysis of the NHS staff survey and outcome data*. 2014.

Shooter, M. Chapter in *Forensic Child and Adolescent Mental Health: Meeting the Needs of Young Offenders.* Edited by Bailey, S., Tarbuck, P. and Chitsabesan, P. 2017.

Young Minds. *#FightingFor Report.* 2018.

Values-Based Child and Adolescent Mental Health System, Commission (2016).

World Health Organization. *Guidelines on optimal feeding of low birth-weight infants in low- and middle-income countries.* 2011.

8

Aligning care in communities

Professor Ilora Baroness Finlay of Llandaff
FRCP, FRCGP, FHEA, FMedSci, FLSW

Baroness Ilora is Professor of Palliative Medicine at Cardiff University and an independent cross-bench member of the House of Lords, where she is also Deputy Speaker. She is President of the Chartered Society for Physiotherapy and Vice President of Hospice UK and of Marie Curie Care.

Wales has a population that is on average slightly older than the rest of the UK and has areas of severe deprivation. For the individual though this often means that children have moved away to find work, leaving the person lonely and potentially isolated when they become frail, but the problem is not confined to the elderly. Young people who become ill or who because of learning difficulties or other problems find themselves needing support, can also be isolated as their own parents become ill themselves or die.

So, what is the answer? Are we to just shrug our shoulders and say we don't have enough resources to go around? Or do we return to the core principles that drove Bevan to address the inequalities so starkly portrayed in the Beveridge report? Do we believe it is an intrinsic scaffolding in society that our autonomy is relational and that we have a duty of care, not only from those paid to care but also from others with whom we interact?

To label those with needs as a burden can be to deny our own humanity, for in giving care we are rewarded by the very act of giving and for the person receiving care there can be an unexpected serenity in receiving. But care can be exhausting and people can feel their generosity is exploited. It is not at all simple.

Compassionate communities

It has been suggested that communities must rediscover their ability to care by harnessing the resources that are there, by organising volunteers and providing them with appropriate support, and by rekindling a sense of interconnectedness. For several decades, political pressures have resulted in calls for more resilience and health promotion activities in communities, but only recently has the concept of co-production extended to a long-standing truth in human relationships – support of each other during difficult times, times of loss, dying, grief and in bereavement. From these rekindled interconnected relationships compassionate communities can emerge.

In those cities and towns where such schemes have been set up, they often are run from the local hospice service, partly because that is a base known and trusted in the community and one with skills at supporting a workforce of volunteers. *An Overview of Compassionate Communities in England* (2013) gathered data on the wide variety of projects that had often built up through the enthusiasm of one or more local champions. It found a need for a clear understanding of the compassionate communities approach in order to disseminate the message and recommended that a supportive environment should be created in order for such activities to thrive and to influence strategic policy in End of Life Care.

Byw Nawr (Live Now) became the Welsh version of Dying Matters. A variety of initiatives developed encouraging people to speak openly about frailty, dying and death itself, to dispel myths about dying and to reconnect people to an awareness of their own mortality.

Why talk about death?

Much health promotion seems aimed at keeping us fit and disease free, with vaccination programmes, tobacco control legislation, moves towards better alcohol control and sporting initiatives. Despite the public health messages, a large proportion of the population lives with chronic conditions, often only moderately controlled. Over time deterioration leads to the inevitable decline to death that is our hallmark – our mortality.

Thanks to medical interventions, death is no longer familiar in the home, it happens behind the doors of institutions: in hospitals, nursing homes and hospices. Reports of the elderly dying on hospital trolleys in overcrowded Emergency Departments have become almost routine, so much so that they are reported in the press with decreasing frequency. Such disrespect of the final phase of a person's life was never envisaged or sanctioned by Bevan. Quite the contrary.

Wales' advantage

Health and Social Care in Wales has not been subjected to the seismic shifts of NHS reorganisation in England. This has allowed continuation of a National service without the silo working promoted by direct competing for NHS England's reforms, which are now inching back towards more integrated accountable care models. When it comes to managing dying, Wales has been ahead of the rest of the world. The *Sugar Report* (2008) set a template for the strategic direction of palliative care services in Wales, the integrated model of a One Wales Palliative Care services has developed.

With representation of and consultation with all stakeholders, core principles of palliative care provision were agreed through co-production ('achieve health and wellbeing with the public, patients and professionals as equal partners through coproduction'), based on the recommendations of the *Sugar Report* which itself took evidence from a wide range of public and professionals. Although the involvement of terminally ill and frail patients was difficult, feedback from relatives and informal feedback via professionals was used to inform the process.

The second prudent healthcare principle underpins the referral guidelines, which set the standard that all urgent referrals should be seen within 48 hours for assessment and instigating appropriate clinical care. Interestingly, wide variation in the way patients are referred has meant that for a significant number of patients, their response to an urgent referral is to ask to defer being seen due to social appointments such as the hairdresser or a family event. Amongst inpatient units the speed of response has meant the standard is almost always met, with Velindre NHS Trust achieving 100% compliance in a recent audit.

A funding formula has ensured services are provided across Wales, consistent with the Prudent Healthcare Principles to 'reduce inappropriate variation using evidence based practices consistently and transparently'. This funding formula has ensured core Specialist Pallative Care (SPC) services are available to populations across Wales using a formula as set out in Table 1. In many areas provision is over and above this thanks to the generous voluntary sector.

Table 1 – Funding formula for the minimum level of
Specialist Palliative Services to be NHS funded

Core staff and whole time equivalents	Area to be covered
One consultant, wherever possible supported by other medical staff	300,000 population community service or 20 hospice beds or 40 cancer centre beds or 850 general hospital beds
One clinical nurse specialist, supporting or supervising other nursing staff	50,000 population or 7 hospice beds or 30 cancer centre beds or 300 general hospital beds (community Clinical Nurse Specialist to link to care homes)
Allied health professions and others	300,000 population for community services
Beds or notional hospice-at-home beds	One per 15,000 population in the community

The upskilling of other services is essential if equitably high standards of care are to be available, as dying patients are ubiquitous across health and social care. A full education programme for primary care, combined with communication skills training, and with national guidelines development in cardiology, nephrology, neurology and respiratory medicine, have aimed to ensure prudent use of professional resources as in Principle 3 'do only what is needed and do no harm, no more, no less'.

The unmet needs of children facing bereavement, whether through the death of a sibling, parent or grandparent, or a close friend or family member must not be ignored. There is powerful evidence that adverse childhood experiences have a devastating effect across a lifetime. This suggests that investment in bereavement support of children is an investment in the long-term wellbeing of our society in Wales, where work with the voluntary sector is establishing a child bereavement coordinator in each Health Board area.

Is need being met?

Across Wales all referrals to specialist palliative care are recorded on the single computerised patient database. The overall number of referrals to these services has risen year-on-year. However, the impact of education programs aimed at primary care and secondary care general providers has resulted in a rise in referral of patients with diagnoses other than cancer and who are in need of palliative care. This has required projects to educate heart failure nurses in cardiac services teams to manage their own palliative problems, developing guidance on the conservative management of renal failure, increasing respiratory support for ventilated patients in the community, targeted support for GPs in managing long-term conditions and is developing, in conjunction with others, appropriate dementia services.

Overall, needs assessment has shown that around two thirds of those patients with palliative care needs are referred at some time for specialist input. The cost effectiveness of this fits with the Welsh health principles as these patients are seen when they need to be seen, the vast majority within 48 hours of an urgent referral, and then deported by the primary care team or other clinical service when an acute complex crisis has been resolved. This speed of response to need is met by the seven day services across Wales, supplemented by 24-hour specialist advice available to health and social care professionals.

Across Wales building initiatives aim to meet the housing needs predicted for the next 10 years and beyond. In these building programmes, a unique opportunity exists to ensure housing is age adaptable, that bathrooms will be suitable, should the occupants become frail, for kitchens to be easily adapted for wheelchair users and that doorways are wide enough to accommodate such requirements. Unfortunately, while planners are required to look at the road schools' infrastructure there is no mandatory requirement that housing is internally adaptable to future requirements. For prudent healthcare to achieve better wellbeing in society, all sectors must be involved.

This also means that community preparedness through dementia friends training is rolled out further. Schools need open conversation to ensure there is support for that the large numbers of children in Wales who have suffered a bereavement (about 10% of our school population, of whom about one third will have lost a parent or sibling). Only through open conversations, sharing emotions and listening to distress will we avoid the results of traumas being handed down generation to generation. The evidence to support a life cycle approach to population wellbeing is powerful, as the outcomes for those who have experienced three or more adverse childhood experiences starkly show. Their health will deteriorate earlier and they will be less resilient to cope with whatever the vagaries of nature and disease throw at them.

In the early stages of frailty

All too often loneliness comes with longevity. As community activities, such as church-going and local high street shopping decline, little has come to replace these points of connectivity between people. Few supermarkets have concurrent activities in their cafes for people to meet around common focus. Many leisure centres have fitness programmes more appropriate to the Lycra wearing than to those needing a walking aid or who have lost social confidence.

Yet there is powerful evidence that input from falls prevention programmes are effective. Those that combine multifactorial assessments with physical movement programmes maintain independence, improve wellbeing and decrease emergency admissions.

On the long road of frailty, even the most devoted family carers can become exhausted. They need looking after and timely respite can give a break and allow them to regain the energy needed. When carers are pushed to breaking point, respite comes too late and is too little to reverse the corrosive effects of exhaustion, feeling unsupported and as if the whole of their lives have become subsumed by caring responsibilities. Respite comes in many guises, from a sitter at home at planned times to admission to a care facility for a fixed planned time to allow carers a break. However, such support is provided there is a golden rule: once promised, the promise must not be broken, because once broken, trust is broken too for the long term. To provide respite needs some more beds in the system. The NHS cannot possibly offer respite, no matter how cost effective in the long term, if it is running at over 90% bed occupancy.

As death approaches – advanced care plans

People know when they are ill, less able to do things for themselves, and they become starkly aware of their own mortality. It is worth then asking why people do not speak more openly, make preparations for the end of life and put their affairs in order. Perhaps it is through fear of making death happen by talking about it, or fear that it is so terrible that a state of denial should be maintained for as long as possible.

This lack of familiarity of death has a lot to answer for. There is a pattern to dying that defies all the horror stories, but is rarely spoken of. Those without pain are extremely unlikely to suddenly get pain, but for everyone the possibility of pain needs to be catered for by anticipatory prescribing. Advance Care Plans must become far more personalised so that they capture a person's wishes and preferences, facilitating open conversations and ensuring that all involved know the anticipated requirements of a person's care. Legal advice or social work involvement can help to 'plan for the worst and hope for the best', by guiding a person to making their will, to considering appointing a trusted person with Lasting Powers of Attorney and to having open conversations with their family.

When dying

As a person becomes weaker, they become more tired, sleeping more on and off and less able to participate in activities. That sleep-wake cycle can slip onwards and instead of sleepiness the person becomes withdrawn and lapses into a coma. From this state their breathing gradually slows, becoming shallower and sometimes irregular until it gently stops. Nothing sudden happens, nothing dramatic, just a gentle slide out of this world.

Throughout these last hours and days family may be there to sit in vigil at the bedside, as they prepare themselves emotionally for the final parting and have the opportunity to say all that they wish they had said before. This is a time for forgiveness, for making amends and for reinforcing bonds of love.

But some people have no family nearby, no close friends who will sit in vigil and watch over their passing. For them a volunteer who will sit with them can be the final and heart-warming sign that our society cares, values the individual and respects the intrinsic worth of each person. The future of care of those nearing the end of life at any age can be transformed by unlocking the goodwill and interpersonal warmth in all communities in Wales. In giving we receive, in receiving we give. Wales can and should rapidly move to become the first Compassionate Country in the world.

References

Murray Hall Community Trust, National Council for Palliative Care & Dying Matters Coalition (2013) *An Overview of Compassionate Communities in England.*
Palliative Care Planning Group Wales (2008) *Report to the Minister for Health and Social Services.*
Byw Nawr - Live Now (Dying Matters in Wales). Available on-line at www.dyingmatters.org/wales

9

What's coming over the hill? Future innovations in medicine and medicines

Professor Philip Routledge CBE

Philip graduated with a Bachelor's degree in Medicine and Surgery (MB BS) in 1972 from the University of Newcastle where he later obtained his MD. He is presently Clinical Director of the All Wales Therapeutics and Toxicology Centre in Cardiff, Emeritus Professor of Clinical Pharmacology at Cardiff University and President Emeritus of the British Pharmacological Society. He was appointed OBE in 2008 and CBE in 2018, both for "Services to Medicine".

Professor Trevor M. Jones CBE FMedSci

Trevor is a former R&D Director of the Wellcome Foundation, a Director of Allergan Inc, the Wales Life Sciences Investment Fund and Director General of The Association of the British Pharmaceutical Industry (ABPI), advisor to UK and EU Governments. He is well known internationally for his activities in clinical research and drug discovery and development in the pharmaceutical industry and has served on many Committees including the UK Government Medicines Commission; Chair of the UK Genetics Advisory Board, the Council of King's College, London and as Commissioner at The World Health Organisation (WHO).

Chris Martin, B Pharm (Hons) FRPharmS

Chris is a pharmacist by profession and currently Deputy Chairman of the Bevan Commission with an interest in Innovation and End of Life care. He has extensive experience in the public sector having been Chairman of four separate health organisations in Wales and until his retirement was the Chairman of Hywel Dda University Health Board, the Welsh NHS Confederation and the co-ordinating chairman of all health organisations in Wales.

He is currently Vice Chairman of the Life Sciences Hub Wales ltd and Non-Executive Director of the Health and Social Services Audit and Risk Committee in Welsh Government. He has several private sector, voluntary and charitable roles including: Chairman MHPA, Board Trustee of Marie Curie UK, Chairman of Wales

Advisory Board for Marie Curie and acts as a mentor on a voluntary and paid basis.

Chris was awarded a fellowship by the Royal Pharmaceutical Society of Great Britain in 2006 for outstanding contribution to the practice of community pharmacy.

Not only was the NHS launched by Aneurin Bevan in 1948 but in that same year, the first randomised controlled clinical trial (of streptomycin in pulmonary tuberculosis) was published by Bradford Hill and colleagues.[1] The increasing rate of drug discovery at this time was assisted by the increased use of randomised controlled clinical trial methodology to rigorously assess the efficacy and safety of these new medicines. The availability of the infrastructure of the newly nationalised health service opened up opportunities to recruit patients to other national clinical trials, resulting in improved therapeutic management of medical conditions. For the next 50 years, pharmaceutical manufacturers, national research bodies and scientists and clinicians worked, often in close collaboration with the NHS, to identify new effective and efficient approaches to the prevention and management of disease.

> *I think Nye Bevan and Sir Austin (Bradford Hill)*
> *have done more for British Medicine than anyone*
> *else in my lifetime.*

Archibald L. Cochrane in *One Man's Medicine* (with Max Blythe) 1989

In 1999, just over 50 years after the founding of the NHS in the UK, the responsibility for the running of NHS in Wales was given to Welsh Government as part of the process of devolution. The first Minister for Health and Social Services, Jane Hutt, set up a Task and Finish Group on Prescribing, chaired by Dr Norman Mills, then Chief Executive of University Hospital

Llandough. One of the Group's main recommendations was that an all-Wales advisory committee should be set up to advise Welsh Government on medicines issues2, and this led to the establishment of the All Wales Medicines Strategy Group (AWMSG) in 2002. Two of the new group's primary roles were to conduct health technology appraisal of selected (usually high-cost) medicines in Wales and to advise Welsh Government on all matters related to prescribing.

Health Technology Appraisal (HTA) in Wales: from "small beginnings"

AWMSG, the first UK HTA group to have its appraisals meetings in public, was initially tasked with advising on the clinical and cost-effectiveness of a relatively small number of new, often high-cost medicines, but this remit was gradually expanded so that AWMSG now appraises all new medicines not on the NICE work programme[3]. In this activity, NICE and AWMSG complement each other and have a joint memorandum of understanding. The goal is to ensure that clinically-effective and cost-effective medicines are made available to patients in Wales as soon as possible. Currently almost 90% of the new medicines appraised by NICE or AWMSG are presently recommended for general use in NHS Wales for either the whole or part of the new licensed indication. The AWMSG HTA processes themselves have been accredited by NICE[4]. AWMSG has also developed its own new approaches to the HTA of medicines for rare diseases (orphan and ultra-orphan medicines) which are designed to take the patient voice more strongly into account[5].

NHS Wales expects that such positively recommended medicines should be included in health board formularies within 30 days of approval and, in association with the introduction of a New Treatment Fund (£80 million over five years), the average time for introduction of NICE or AWMSG-approved new medicines to health board formularies has fallen to 10 days over the first 12 months of the Fund's existence[6]. Wales did not follow England in introducing a Cancer Drugs Fund, preferring not to prioritise one specific medical condition (cancer) over all others. Despite this, there was evidence that some recently-launched cancer medicines which were subsequently recommended by NICE were adopted faster in Wales than in England[7].

Prudent prescribing as part of the prudent healthcare agenda in Wales

Prudent healthcare is "healthcare which is conceived, managed and delivered in a cautious and wise way characterised by forethought, vigilance and careful budgeting which achieves tangible benefits and quality outcomes for patients". The frequency of multi-morbidity (having more than one medical condition concurrently) has increased as people in Wales and elsewhere in the UK enjoy higher life expectancy. Multi-morbidity brings with it an increased incidence of polypharmacy, sometimes appropriate but also at times inappropriate or 'problematic' as a result of imprudent healthcare.[8] Polypharmacy may lead to an increased risk of adverse drug events, including drug-drug interactions and medication errors. Some of these situations may result in medicines-related admissions, and at any one time, it has been estimated that around 230 hospital beds are occupied by patients who have been admitted as a result of adverse reactions to medicines.[9]

In 2014, AWMSG produced guidance on prescribing in polypharmacy situations[10] and this was reinforced in 16 targeted, well-received case-based prudent prescribing workshops across Wales in 2014/15, using materials based on the All Wales National Prescribing Indicators (NPIs).[11] NPIs have been used in Wales since AWMSG introduced them (selected by national consensus) in 2002. They are generally measures of the efficiency and/or quality of prescribing and they allow benchmarking between prescribers, practices, GP clusters and health boards in Wales or further afield. If collected over a period of time, they are can identify changing trends in what is being prescribed (or more accurately, dispensed), but not why any observed changes might have occurred.

In 2014/15 all NPIs moved in the desired direction in association with the delivery of the prudent prescribing workshop programme except for the total volume of antibiotic prescribing in Wales.[12] However, desired reductions were seen in that year in the NPIs measuring proportional use of some antibiotic groups defined by WHO as "critically important antibiotics (CIAs)" such as quinolones, cephalosporins and co-amoxiclav (all as a % of total antibacterial items). Then in 2015/16 the total volume of antibiotic prescribing in Wales began to fall for the first time and has fallen further again in 2016/17.[13]

The second prudent healthcare principle is to "care for those with the greatest health need first, making the most effective use of all skills and resources". In 2001, Wales was the first country to decide to phase out prescription "co-payments", which were eventually fully abolished in 2007. The aim was to improve health through removal of possible barriers to patients in Wales (particularly those with low income) taking all the medicines they had been prescribed. A recent study indicated that during the phased abolition, dispensing in Wales did show a small but significant increase in 14 pre-selected medicines (those which had the highest percentage of items dispensed subject to a co-payment prior to abolition) compared with the north east of England, an area with very similar health and socio-economic characteristics to Wales but where prescription co-payments continued during the study period.[14] Northern Ireland subsequently adopted a free-prescription policy in 2010 and Scotland in 2011. Such natural experiments illustrate the value of comparing different approaches in the different UK nations to inform the development of new health policies, including those involving medicines.

HTA in 2018 and beyond: What's on the horizon?

After a relatively slow start, personalised (precision) medicine is increasingly contributing to the effective and efficient treatment of important medical conditions. Several clinically useful biomarkers are now in general use and can identify those individuals most likely to benefit from the treatment or those most likely to be at risk of side effects. The genomics strategy for Wales describes how Wales will move forward in this area, recognising that it is vital to work with the people of Wales to "support the development of an open, transparent and publicly agreed approach to the sharing of genomic and precision medicine data for service development and research."[15]

Cell and gene therapy, also referred to as regenerative medicine, has the potential to address unmet need for treatment (and sometimes possibly cure) in certain areas of unmet need. Such medicines may be extremely expensive, but nevertheless confer major benefits. A large budget impact allied to possible uncertainty around relative benefits and risks in the early stages of use may delay the rate of uptake of these products, so new innovative approaches to reimbursement may well be required in future to achieve early market access.[16]

Not all advances in therapeutics involve medicines. The Health Technology Hub for Wales is now delivering a coordinated approach to the identification, appraisal and adoption of new non-medicine technologies. It is working to build a strong partnership between academic bodies and healthcare organisations such as the NHS Wales Informatics Service and the new appraisal body, Health Technology Wales has already commenced its work-programme for non-medicine technologies.

The future of prudent prescribing as part of the prudent healthcare challenge

The NHS in Wales is faced with the need to improve health and drive forward an efficient and equitable health and social care system in the context of an ageing population, increasing demand and financial constraints. These same issues are also major challenges for other healthcare systems within the UK and internationally. AWMSG has thus already endorsed the proposals for disinvestment outlined in *Medicines Identified as Low Priority for Funding in NHS Wales* thereby seeking to release resources in order to re-invest in more clinically- and cost-effective alternatives[17].

The third prudent healthcare principle is "do only what is needed, no more, no less; and do no harm." The AWMSG Strategy for 2018-2023[18] aims to align with the goal of the World Health Organization (WHO) Global Patient Safety Challenge, Medication without Harm, to reduce the level of severe, avoidable harm in Wales over the next five years.[19]

Bevan Fellows and the Prudent Pharmacy

Several pharmacists have now been Bevan Exemplars in the first two Bevan Academy cohorts, often working in in multidisciplinary teams to undertake academic studies of prudent healthcare delivery. They have contributed to valuable projects on reducing medicines waste in care homes, medicines reconciliation, more efficient home dialysis delivery, improved antimicrobial stewardship, avoidance of medicine-associated gastrointestinal bleeding and healthcare associated infections.[20,21] More pharmacists will be encouraged to apply for future Exemplar cohorts or to become Bevan Fellows and be able to support prudent healthcare developments in Wales.

Figure 1 – Integrated Pharmacy Services – wrapping around the patient[24]

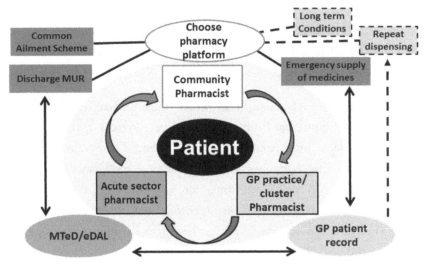

MUR = Medicines Use Review; MTeD = Medicines Transcribing and e-Discharge, an electronic means of recording a list of medications for a patient and adding them to an electronic discharge advice letter (e-DAL). The e-DAL is then sent to the patient's GP as soon as they leave the ward, via the Welsh Clinical Communications Gateway.

Community pharmacies and the pharmacists who work in them have a pivotal role to play in supporting the outworking of prudent health and care within local communities.

The concept of the "Prudent Pharmacy" begins by identifying the needs of local people in order to help them manage chronic conditions as well as minor ailments, and when possible avoid unnecessary visits to GP and other healthcare services. There are over 700 community pharmacies in Wales, with the highest numbers in deprived population areas where the need is greatest. The introduction in Wales of the 'Choose Pharmacy' (now known as Common Ailments) formulary in a pilot programme was associated with a reduction in the number of prescriptions issued by GPs, and national roll-out may achieve even greater savings.[13,22]

In 2018/19, the Wales Centre for Postgraduate Pharmacy Education (WCPPE) will be working with the All Wales Therapeutics and Toxicology Centre (AWTTC) to produce educational resources for community pharmacists based around prudent prescribing and the NPIs. These resources will support community pharmacists when they conduct medicines use reviews (MURs) with patients.

The importance of digital technologies

Virtually all of the new developments and initiatives in therapeutics described above are to a greater or lesser extent dependent upon the availability of data and information resources, a vital component clearly outlined by the Parliamentary Review of Health and Social Care in Wales.[23] Assistive technologies, artificial intelligence and technology-enabled care initiatives (e.g. telemedicine and telecare) will have a major role to play in the future efficient delivery of health and social care and companies. A new digital health ecosystem has been created to help technology companies access health and care sector platforms and share digital health innovations. Electronic prescribing has been enormously important in primary care and will be equally important as soon as it is introduced into the secondary care (hospital) sector in Wales.[18]

Conclusions

For 70 years the Health Service has continued to be the means by which comprehensive, effective and efficient healthcare is available to the public free at the point of use, adhering to the fundamental principles first outlined in the White Paper "A National Health Service" in 1944. Huge strides have been made in introducing innovative medicines and other treatments to the NHS since the service was launched in 1948. However, the Parliamentary Review of Health and Social Care in Wales highlights the pressing future challenge to further "harness innovation and accelerate technology and infrastructure developments" in order to deliver more effective and efficient care, clear health outcomes and value for money for the people of Wales.[23]

References

1. Medical Research Council Streptomycin in Tuberculosis Trials Committee. *Streptomycin treatment for pulmonary tuberculosis*. Br med J 1948; 2: 735-746. https://www.ncbi.nlm.nih.gov/pmc/articles/PMC2091872/

2. National Assembly for Wales. *Report of the Task and Finish Group on Prescribing* 2000 www.assembly.wales/Committee%20Documents/HSS-05-01(p.1)%20%20Report%20of%20the%20Task%20and%20Finish%20Group%20on%20Prescribing-14032001-30405/3aa76ed9000bf0480000606200000000-English.pdf#search=Task%20Finish%20Prescribing (Accessed 26 April 2018)

3. Varnava A, Bracchi R, Samuels K, Hughes DA, Routledge PA. *New Medicines in Wales: The All Wales Medicines Strategy Group (AWMSG) Appraisal Process and Outcomes. Pharmacoeconomics.* 2018 Mar 8. doi: 10.1007/s40273-018-0632-7. [Epub ahead of print] https://link.springer.com/article/10.1007%2Fs40273-018-0632-7 (Accessed 26 April 2018)

4. National Institute for Health and Care Excellence. *NICE accreditation decisions.* All Wales Medicines Strategy Group. 2016. https://www.nice.org.uk/About/ What-we-do/Accreditation/ Accreditation-decisions (Accessed 17 March 2018)

5. All Wales Medicines Strategy Group. *Policy for appraising orphan and ultra-orphan medicines, and medicines developed for rare diseases – feedback from the pilot.* http://www.awmsg.org/awmsgonline/app/sitesearch;jsessionid= 38844a15989ba1823e07270c40ce?execution=e1s1 (Accessed 26 April 2018)

6. *New drugs access 'faster than ever'* - Welsh Government. BBC News 23/01/2018. http://www.bbc.co.uk/news/uk-wales-42775136 (Accessed 26 April 2018)

7. Chamberlain C, Collin SM, Stephens P, Donovan J, Bahl A, Hollingworth W. *Does the cancer drugs fund lead to faster uptake of cost-effective drugs? A time-trend analysis comparing England and Wales.* Br J Cancer.2014 Oct 28;111(9):1693-702. doi: 10.1038/bjc.2014.86. Epub 2014 Feb 25. https://www.ncbi.nlm.nih.gov/pmc/articles/PMC4453744/ (Accessed 26 April 2018)

8. Routledge P. A. *Better health outcomes and safer care through prudent prescribing.* http://www.prudenthealthcare.org.uk/prescribing/ (Accessed 26 April 2018)

9. Auditor General for Wales. *Managing medicines in primary and secondary care.* Wales Audit Office, December 2016. https://www.wao.gov.uk/system/files/ publications/Medicines-management-2016-english.pdf (Accessed 26 April 2018)

10. All Wales Medicines Strategy Group. *Polypharmacy: Guidance for Prescribing.* 2014. http://www.awmsg.org/awmsgonline/app/sitesearch?execution=e1s1 (Accessed 26 April 2018)

11. Hayes J., Bracchi R., Collier C., Coulson J. M., Deslandes P., Jones K., Haines K.E., Jenkins K., Lewis T., Snooks J., Wilkins S., Routledge P. A. *Prudent Prescribing Workshops to support the Prudent Healthcare agenda in Wales in 2014-15.* http://www.pa2online.org/ (Accessed 26 April 2018)

12. Haines K. E., Coulson J. M., Jenkins K., Howard-Baker L., Jones K., Deslandes P., Lewis T., Bracchi R., Hayes J., Samuels K., Routledge P. A.. *The role of nationally agreed Prescribing Indicators (NPIs) in promoting Prudent Prescribing as part of Prudent Healthcare in Wales.* http://www.pa2online.org/ (Accessed 26 April 2017)

13. All Wales Medicines Strategy Group. Annual report 2016-17. http://www.awmsg.org/docs/awmsg/awmsgdocs/AWMSG%20Annual%20Repor t%202016%20-%202017.pdf (Accessed 26 April 2018)

14. Alam M. F., Cohen D., Dunstan F., Hughes D., Routledge P. *Impact of the phased abolition of co-payments on the utilisation of selected prescription medicines in Wales. Health Econ.* 2018 Jan;27(1):236-243. doi: 10.1002/hec.3530. Epub 2017 Jul 7. https://onlinelibrary.wiley.com/doi/abs/10.1002/hec.3530 (Accessed 26 April 2018)

15. Welsh Government. http://gov.wales/docs/dhss/publications/170802genomics-straten.pdf (Accessed 26 April 2017)

16. Kefalos P. *Cell and Gene therapy Reimbursement: the CGC Approach.* 2016. https://ct.catapult.org.uk/sites/default/files/The-Cell-and-Gene-Therapy-Catapult-approach-to-pricing-and-reimbursement-strategy-development.pdf (Accessed 26 April 2017)

17. All Wales Medicines Strategy Group. *Medicines Identified as Low Priority for Funding in NHS Wales.* http://www.awmsg.org/docs/awmsg/medman/Medicines%20Identified%20as%20Low%20Priority%20for%20Funding%20in%20NHS%20Wales.pdf (Accessed 26 April 2018)

18. All Wales Medicines Strategy Group. *Five-year Strategy 2018-2023.* http://www.awmsg.org/docs/awmsg/awmsgdocs/AWMSG%20Five%20Year%20Strategy%202018-2023.pdf (Accessed 26 April 2018)

19. World Health Organization. *Medication without harm – WHO Global Patient Safety Challenge.* May 2017. http://www.who.int/patientsafety/medication-safety/en/ (Accessed 26 April 2017)

20. Bevan Academy for Leadership & Innovation 2016/17 Exemplar Showcase http://www.bevancommission.org/publications?start=5&count=5&d=1 (Accessed 26 April 2017)

21. Bevan Commission Academy Innovators. http://www.bevancommission.org/publications?start=5&count=5&d=1 (Accessed 26 April 2018)

22. All Wales Medicines Strategy Group. *All Wales Common Ailments Formulary.* http://www.awmsg.org/awmsgonline/app/sitesearch;jsessionid=a616d421233cc9e330134443d251?execution=e1s1 (Accessed 26 April 2018)

23. The Parliamentary Review of Health and Social Care in Wales. https://beta.gov.wales/sites/default/files/publications/2018-01/Review-health-social-care-report-final.pdf (Accessed 26 April 2018)

24. Scott-Thomas, S. (2018). *Personal Communication*

10

Working life and
health inequality

Professor Dame Carol Black DBE, FRCP, FMedSci

Dame Carol is Principal of Newnham College Cambridge and Expert Adviser on Health and Work to NHS England and Public Health England. She is a past-President of the Royal College of Physicians, of the Academy of Medical Royal Colleges, and of the British Lung Foundation, and past-Chair of the Nuffield Trust for health policy. She chairs the Board of Think Ahead, the Government's new fast-stream training programme for Mental Health Social Workers, and the RSSB's Health and Wellbeing Policy Group. She was a member of the Welsh Government's Parliamentary Review of Health and Social Care in Wales the board of UK Active, Rand Europe's Council of Advisers, PwC's Health Industries Oversight Board, and the Advisory Board of Step up to Serve.

As many have shown, most recently my fellow Bevan Commissioner Sir Michael Marmot, numerous factors underlie inequalities in health. Such inequalities affect life chances and working life. Impaired working life can have adverse impacts on the health and wellbeing not only of the individuals affected but also on their families and on the community at large.

Work itself affects health and wellbeing. There are economic, social and moral arguments that good work is the most effective way to improve the wellbeing of individuals, their families and their communities. There is also growing awareness that long-term worklessness is harmful to physical and mental health.

For these reasons a major challenge is to enable and support people who are not wholly fit and well to enter and maintain fulfilling working lives. Moreover, as a consequence of demographic changes and increasing life expectancy, part of that challenge is to enable people to extend their working lives beyond the traditional point called retirement.

Safeguarding and promoting the health and wellbeing of the people of working age in Wales; minimising the risk of illness including risks arising from the working environment; and supporting rehabilitation of those who become ill or disabled, enabling them to maintain, resume or take up work; are all major components of the public health endeavour.

These actions have a necessary part in achieving an overarching aim of reducing health inequalities. To minimise demands upon a precarious economy it has become even more important to keep people fit and in work, and so reduce the social and economic burdens of sickness – especially long-term sickness – and loss of work and loss of productivity.

I am clear that the workplace has a major role in protecting and promoting health. This includes a part in addressing the major problems surrounding mental health and in supporting people with long term disorders, enabling as many people as to fulfil their potential in the workplace. It means establishing a strong cultural lead and example in organisations, and strengthening management training to recognise and respond to the health needs of the workforce; and working more closely with other health supporting agencies, particularly occupational health and primary care.

Enlightened employers recognise the importance of shaping a workplace culture in which supporting and safeguarding the health and wellbeing of all members of the workforce has high priority. It is important that this culture permeates other organisations and becomes the norm not only in Wales but further afield.

Welsh government policy and health indicators

Since devolution Welsh Government has produced healthcare policy which has contributed to a divergent policy landscape in Wales compared to the rest of the UK. There is a recurring discourse of development and improvement associated with WG health policies, often framed by terms such as fairer, better, or a more equal Wales. The focus on such goals to improve however belies the complexity of their realisation in Wales.

These successive policies are indeed aspirational when we consider that Wales is disproportionately burdened in comparison to the rest of the UK in terms of chronic illness, social deprivation and a legacy of ill health spanning several generations. It has been suggested that persistent health inequalities have been ever present in Wales for at least 150 years, essentially since data first existed and have been recorded (CMO, 2011).

Recent National surveys in Wales (2017) have shown that 47% of adults reported they had a physical or mental health condition or illness which was expected to last for 12 months or more. Furthermore 33% stated they had a condition or illness which limited their ability to carry out day-to-day tasks.

While there have been improvements in some health indicators in Wales these are broadly similar to those achieved in other areas of the UK. This means that Wales will have to continually over perform in the areas with the greatest deficit to make up ground within the UK and to ultimately deliver healthcare outcomes that are 'world class'.

The working Welsh population

While England has had higher total population growth, Wales has experienced a greater growth in its older population. This is matched by a corresponding decrease in the youngest age group with Wales experiencing a 5.4% decline in the number of under-14s between 2001 and 2011. It is unsurprising therefore that the healthcare workforce in Wales is also ageing, with 1 in 3 staff aged over 50 (NSSP, 2015).

There is a well-recognised loss of young people from Wales, for example school leavers who attend Universities outside of Wales many of whom choose never to return, representing a reduction of human, social and cultural capital (Wyn Jones, 2012). This is unsurprising given the perceived benefits of migrating from Wales, such as better quality jobs, more opportunities in the private sector and higher earnings, reflecting the relative lack of similar opportunities for graduates who remain (Bristow et al., 2011).

The main source of good quality employment in Wales remains the public sector, which employs approximately half of post-1992 young graduates who were born and live there. The most recent employment rate in Wales (WG, 2018) estimates 72.6% of those aged 16-64 were in work, lower than the equivalent UK figure (75.3%).

It is often assumed that a healthy workforce means a healthy economy, yet how health impacts on income is often controversial (Fritters et al., 2005). Conventional measures to improve productivity, from investment in skills, technology and innovation to labour market deregulation, fail to take account of one of the most serious barriers to growing prosperity: poor workforce health (Bevan, 2014).

The causes of sickness absence and poor performance are most commonly around health problems (stress / anxiety / mild depression), musculoskeletal problems (back / neck / shoulder / arm pain) and the quality of work / workplace (leadership / managerial behaviour and board engagement). Other important reasons include long-term conditions and social issues within the home and a lack of education and/or skills. These reasons why we don't go to work can cause people to lose their jobs quickly but they are things we could and should change.

Deprivation in Wales

Wales is generally regarded as having a relatively poor health status, coupled with relatively high levels of deprivation. Deprivation clusters in Wales, particularly around former industrial areas (Figure 1) where levels of economic activity are low with pockets of inter-generational worklessness. Multiple deprivations often stop people from finding and being in work and this is the same across the regions of the UK (Aylward and Phillips, 2008).

The impact of social factors upon health, mediated as Marmot says through causes of causes, is vividly and decisively confirmed in the gradient of measures of ill health against degrees of deprivation (Figure 1).

Mental health is one of the commonest reasons for not being in work and is often found to be more likely in deprived areas (Figure 2). Businesses and institutions need to recognise that

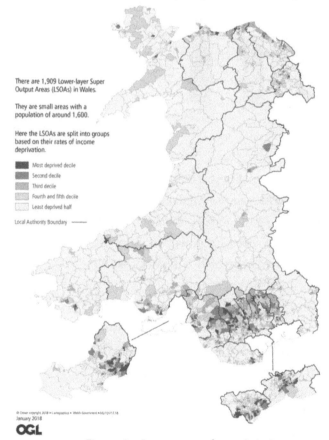

There are 1,909 Lower-layer Super Output Areas (LSOAs) in Wales.

They are small areas with a population of around 1,600.

Here the LSOAs are split into groups based on their rates of income deprivation.

■ Most deprived decile
■ Second decile
▨ Third decile
▧ Fourth and fifth decile
▢ Least deprived half

Local Authority Boundary ——

© Crown copyright 2018 • Cartographica • Welsh Government • MJ/10317.18
January 2018

OGL

Figure 1 – Percentage of people in income deprivation, lower-layer super output areas of Wales 2016-17.

mental health is a business issue. While the economic cost of absence due to mental health is high, the human cost can be far higher. Managers need help to understand it, and be appropriately trained. Sadly, it is often the case poor leadership or management and the reaction to it contributes to ill-health.

Figure 2 – Percentage of adults who reported being treated for any mental illness, by deprivation quintile

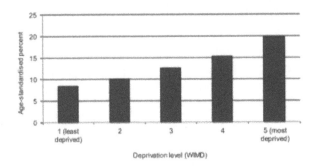

There is a 10-fold difference in Incapacity Benefit rates between the least and most deprived communities in local authorities across England and Wales (Waddell and Aylward, 2010). In Wales 11.6% of the 16-64 population are in receipt of income benefit (Job Seekers Allowance, Employment Support Allowance & Incapacity Benefit and Lone Parent) which is higher that all English regions except the north east (12.2%) (StatsWales, 2016).

An ideal benefits system has two chief purposes: to ensure that personal needs are compassionately, carefully and promptly assessed, to ensure appropriate and timely award of benefits; and to also assess and provide the necessary healthcare, social support and occupational health and employment support to enable the best possible employment.

We need to look more at the 'causes of causes' to understand how we might be able to begin to change the historical patterns and impact of deprivation. The clear adverse effects of deprivation and poor educational opportunity begin before individuals enter their working lives. This is then further compounded by often starting in poor-quality jobs with little opportunity to progress and with compounding effects on health and persisting inequalities.

The NHS workforce

The current NHS workforce in Wales is made up of approximately 89, 000 people by headcount or 76,288 by full time equivalent (FTE). The difference between headcount and FTE is a useful indicator of the prevalence of part-time staff in the NHS workforce. This represents around 4.5% of the 16-64 age group in Wales, although this varies by welsh region from 3 to 16% (NHS Welsh Confed., 2015). Any new policy approaches that impacts on healthcare workforce redesign can therefore have a disproportionate social effect in such areas where so many look to the NHS for employment in Wales, in comparison to countries with more diverse economies.

Staff absence due to sickness is approximately 5% in the NHS Wales workforce Welsh Government (2017). The Welsh Ambulance Services NHS Trust had the highest sickness absence (6.4%) of all NHS Wales organisations and has done so since data started to be collected in 2008. These absence rates are higher than those seen in the general workforce in Wales which the ONS reports to be around 2.6% (ONS, 2017). However, this figure is the highest for any region in the UK and means that the Wales suffers most from days lost to sickness.

The Parliamentary Review into Health and Care

The final report of the Parliamentary Review into Health and Care (2018) in Wales highlighted that "Wales needs a different system of care" and made 10 key recommendations. The future vision for this system 'must articulate a clear and simple vision of what care will look like in the future, organised around the individual and their family as close to home as possible – it should be preventative with easy access and of high quality, in part enabled via digital technology, delivering what users and the wider public say really matters to them. Furthermore, care and support should be seamless, without artificial barriers between physical and mental health, primary and secondary care, or health and social care'.

As part of recommendation 5, 'A great place to work', which focused on the future health and care workforce, a number of supportive actions were proposed. These included many well recognised approaches such as; the need for joint work force planning at regional level; deliver staff with new skills and integrated career paths; joined up approach to recruitment across all areas; and a clear focus on improving and maintain the health and wellbeing of the current workforce. There was however little challenge in the way of new or novel holistic roles or approaches and detailed reference to the impact of technology in the future.

What can be done in Wales?

In economic and social terms our ability to meet society's service needs and expectations, including our capacity to support dependants – children, pensioners, and the unemployed – depends on the productivity of those who are in employment. Through our work to date the Bevan Commission has recognised the complexity and impact of wide ranging factors affecting health and wellbeing which include education, employment, housing and skills and the everyday living and working environment.

We have recognised the importance of maintaining workability and independence in an ageing population and that the wider public sector should have a more common purpose; that of enabling people to do as much as possible for as long as possible, or as long as they want in both their working and personal lives.

Most significant has been the development of Prudent Healthcare (Bevan Commission, 2014) and its underlying principles which aim to respond to the complex interconnected challenges facing healthcare systems both in Wales and elsewhere. In addition, the development of a prudent social model for health through its Heritage Paper series has articulate what the future of health and care delivery should look like and the importance of the workforce in delivering this.

Society needs the maximum number of productive years from as many people as possible. Those who are not working depend on others. We need to work longer, we are living longer. If we are going to have a welfare state we need enough workers to provide for the needy. We need the ratio of earners and wealth-generators to dependants (children, pensioners, and the unemployed) to be as high as possible. Being sufficiently healthy is a condition for work, and maximising healthy life as a proportion of total life is therefore a desirable goal for individuals and society.

The recent Parliamentary review of which I was a member asked that if the case for change in Wales is so compelling, then why hasn't it compelled? I would think just as equally compelling is to ask how much longer will Wales tolerate such differences in health, wellbeing and inequality?

References

Aylward M. A. & Phillips G. (2008). *Report for Edwina Hart AM MBE, Minister for Health and Social Services*. Welsh Assembly Government.

Bevan Commission. (2014). Prudent Healthcare Principles.

Bevan S. et al. (2014). *Fit for work: Musculoskeletal disorders in the European Workforce*. The Work Foundation.

Bristow, G. et al. (2011). *Stay, leave or return? Patterns of Welsh graduate mobility*. People, Place & Policy Online. 5(3): p. 135-148.

Chief Medical Officer for Wales. (2011). *Our Healthy Future: Annual Report 2011*. Welsh Government.

Frijters, P. et al. (2005). *The causal effect of income on health: evidence from German reunification. Journal of Health Economics* 24, 997–1017.

Marmot, M. (2008). *Closing the gap in a generation: Health equity through action on the social determinants of health*

NWSSP (2015). *NHS Wales Workforce Age Profile 2015*.

Office for National statistics. (2017). *Sickness absence in the labour market: 2016*.

StatsWales (2016*) Benefit claimants by Welsh local authority and statistical group*

Parliamentary Review into Health and Care. (2018). *Final Report*. Welsh Government.

Waddell G. & Aylward M. A. (2010). *Models of sickness and disability applied to common health problems*.

Welsh Economic Review (2012*). Interview with Professor Richard Wyn Jones*. p. 22-24.

Welsh Government (2017). *Sickness absence in the NHS in Wales, quarter ended 30 June 2017*

Welsh NHS Confederation. (2015) *From Rhetoric to Reality – NHS Wales in 10 years' time; The NHS Wales Workforce*.

11

The role of industry and technology in creating a prudent society

Professor Trevor M. Jones CBE FMedSci

Trevor is a former R&D Director of the Wellcome Foundation, a Director of Allergan Inc, the Wales Life Sciences Investment Fund and Director General of The Association of the British Pharmaceutical Industry (ABPI), advisor to UK and EU Governments. He is well known internationally for his activities in clinical research and drug discovery and development in the pharmaceutical industry and has served on many Committees including the UK Government Medicines Commission; Chair of the UK Genetics Advisory Board, the Council of King's College, London and as Commissioner at The World Health Organisation (WHO).

Wales is home to a thriving and expanding Life Sciences Industry with over 250 companies employing over 15,000 people involved in a broad range of products from the discovery and development of new medicines, including clinical research through the development of specialised medical equipment, to the manufacture of Diagnostics and Medicines.

Across Wales there are both large international companies such as technology specialists GE Healthcare, Siemens, Renishaw, pharmaceutical companies such as Norgine, Ipsen UK Ltd and Wockhardt as well as local companies such as PCI, Protherics UK Ltd, Calon Cardio Technology, Sphere Medical ReNeuron, Synexus and Simbec-Orion. In addition, most of the world's largest pharmaceutical companies, such as GlaxoSmithKline, AstraZeneca, Pfizer and Roche have active collaborations across Wales, working with healthcare professionals and supplying prescription and pharmacy medicines to the NHS.

In fact, Wales has 5% of the UK population but 10% of its life sciences workforce and can rightly claim to have the UK's most successful cluster of in-vitro diagnostic companies. These include Ortho Clinical Diagnostics, Quotient Bioresearch, Quay and AMRI. Larval therapy firm, ZooBiotic, now dominates the world market in such products (having been the first spin-out from an NHS Trust).

As well as making a significant contribution to the health and wealth of Wales, these companies provide employment to sustain both individuals and their families and support to their neighbouring communities. Although the primary function of the life sciences industry is to manage successful businesses, they recognise that they share a common commitment to improve the lives of the people of Wales, working alongside healthcare professionals and patients. Through such partnerships, these companies learn which aspects of their businesses are most relevant to the health and wellbeing of people in Wales and in return share their special knowledge and expertise with those directly involved in the day-to-day delivery of healthcare.

The organisation that represents pharmaceutical companies in Wales, The

Association of the British Pharmaceutical Industry Wales (ABPI Wales) and its members work in partnership with the National Assembly for Wales, Welsh Government, NHS Wales, patient organisations and other key stakeholders, to help address the health needs of the people of Wales. This includes being active participants in strategic NHS organisations, such as the All Wales Diabetes Implementation Group and Heart Conditions Implementation Group and other groups supporting developments in Wales, including Respiratory Alliance Wales (RAW), the Welsh Respiratory Innovation Centre Working Group, Cancer Cross-Party Group and most recently the Cell and Gene Therapy Task and Finish Group under the leadership of the Welsh Blood Service.

At a time when funding for health, healthcare and wellbeing is stretched, the pharmaceutical industry in Wales is committed to working with Government and the NHS to deliver value for money from medicines, better patient access to medicines and to ensure innovation and research are rewarded. In particular, and in line with the Bevan Prudent Principles, this includes the generation of best practice, 'holistic' commissioning leading to better patient outcomes, developing outcomes frameworks... including patient reported outcome measures... and the co-creation of measures to drive adoption and uptake of innovative medicines.

It is important that the actions of these companies are linked to the need of the people of Wales and not solely to the commercial benefit of the industry.

ABPI Wales has outlined a number of key principles relating to partnerships with patients, the public, healthcare professionals and government viz:

- Patients must be at the heart of the future NHS, with patient choice, access to medicines and patient outcomes as the key pillars of success.

- A culture that embraces innovation, including swift adoption of best practice, must be truly embedded within the whole health and social care system.

- Active engagement of all stakeholders, including the pharmaceutical industry, is vital at all levels of NHS Wales. Degrees of stakeholder engagement should be measured and built into the constitutions of all decision-making bodies, from the local level through to strategic bodies like the All Wales Medicines Strategy Group (AWMSG).

- All processes must be transparent, consistent and translatable to all levels and locations of the NHS.

- Bureaucracy should be minimised at all levels, with particular emphasis on not duplicating decisions at local levels, to facilitate rapid uptake of innovative medicines.

- Accountability at all levels of the health system must be clear and transparent to ensure implementation of decisions and avoid, and tackle if necessary, any system failures.

- The pharmaceutical industry should be seen as a valuable partner rather than simply a supplier of medicines.

There are recent collaborative projects that demonstrate how these partnerships can work successfully. For example, the overarching aim of the Diabetes Research Unit Cymru (DRU Cymru) at Swansea Singleton Campus is to support a comprehensive, integrated translational research programme, designed to advance development and implementation of therapeutic strategies for prevention and treatment of diabetes.

The unit recently carried out a collaborative study on Diabetes with The Bevan Commission and Janssen Pharmaceuticals. The study used the SAIL Database at Swansea University to examine the health outcomes of all people diagnosed with Diabetes in Wales between 1999-2014; looking at the type of prescription medicine they were taking, variations in disease control: age, gender and deprivation.

They found that time and age of diagnosis seems to be the biggest factor in poor diabetes control. Also, that diabetes is more prevalent in deprived areas and that poor health was related to delays between poor control and increased medication use. These findings are leading to improvement in diagnosis, monitoring and treatment so improving the lives and, importantly, the employment of patients, their families and carers and the prudent use of scarce healthcare resource.

It is critically important that companies work closely in partnership with patients, patient organisations, communities and third sector organisations. Such collaborative partnerships are not restricted to the pharmaceutical sector but involve other life science companies.

MediWales is an organisation that was established to encourage such joint workings in Wales and to provide advice, support and business opportunities for its members. It is an independent, not-for-profit organisation that has a network of 180 members largely made up of life science organisations, pharmaceutical services and medical technology companies. It actively encourages engagement with the clinical research community and membership includes NHS health boards and universities.

Access to clinical expertise is an essential part of the product development process for medical devices and pharmaceuticals, so MediWales collaborates regularly with the NHS, and academic and research groups to facilitate industry access to appropriate clinical expertise.

As with health and wellbeing in the community, funding innovation is a key determinant of growing a successful future for the people of Wales. The Welsh Government recognised this need and created a dedicated £100m Life Sciences Fund. It has world-leading academic expertise, a talent-drawing £50m initiative and a central Life Sciences Hub.

Arthurian Life Sciences was given the remit of managing the fund and making Wales an attractive destination for UK and international companies operating in the sector.

Built on an initial investment of £45m, the WLSIF has:

- Created a portfolio of 10 investments;
- Delivered an internal rate of return (IRR) of 26% (3-year IRR at 31 March 2016);
- Attracted £380m UK and international co-investment;
- Created 150 high-tech and highly skilled jobs and aims to create a further 200 jobs; and
- Established a portfolio of 23 highly valuable therapeutic products and medical devices currently under development for stroke, cancer, blindness, respiratory disease, vascular disease, cystic fibrosis and diabetes.

One such example is the establishment of a cancer centre in Newport by Proton Partners International. This centre is at the vanguard of advancing cancer care in the UK. The centre will provide an all-encompassing cancer service, delivering high energy proton beam therapy, imaging, chemotherapy, radiotherapy, immunotherapy and a range of supportive care services.

Proton beam therapy is a highly-targeted type of radiotherapy that can treat hard-to-reach cancers, such as spinal tumours, with a lower risk of damaging the surrounding tissue and causing side effects.

The centre, in Newport, is the first in the UK to have Proton Beam technology so enabling patients in Wales to be first to gain benefit from this state of the art technology.

NHS Wales recognises the importance of obtaining objective evidence that treatments are both clinically and, importantly, cost effective. At the heart of this is the conduct of clinical trials where Wales is well placed with the expertise in its hospitals, general practices and Clinical Research Organisations (CRO's) such as Simbec-Orion and Synexus as well as University/NHS based centres of excellence such as the Centre for Trials Research Cardiff University, The Clinical Research and Innovation Centre at the Aneurin Bevan University Health Board, the Early Phase Unit at Velindre Cancer Centre (Cardiff) and the Clinical Research Unit (CRU) in the Institute for Life Sciences at Swansea University.

Indeed, many international pharmaceutical companies are now funding clinical research in these CRO companies and in the NHS in Wales.

In that context, Vaughan Gething AM, Cabinet Secretary for Health and Social Services made an announcement during a visit in July 2017 to the Clinical Research and Innovation Centre at Aneurin Bevan University Health Board that the Welsh Government will invest more than £21m during 2018 in high quality research in the Welsh NHS to help researchers develop the treatments for tomorrow. He said "We want to make Wales one of the most attractive places in the world for academic and clinical research... which will help attract the best talent to Wales."

The emphasis on clinical research in Wales has been strengthened through the establishment of Health and Care Research Wales (formerly NISCHR) which, in consultation with partners, develops policy on research and development to reflect the health and social care priorities of the Welsh Government. It delivers its strategy and policies through commissioning services, running research schemes and initiatives, and through strategic investment and partnership working with other funding bodies, the NHS, academia, industry and other key partners.

It has a clearly stated strategy (from 2012) for Industry Engagement in Wales viz:

- For the NHS to play a pivotal role in delivering research, development and innovation and develop a business-friendly culture where engagement with industry is a core organisational activity.
- For engagement between academia and industry to become a natural process of innovative collaboration which results in addressing unmet clinical needs and economic growth.
- For Wales based researchers to play a greater role in securing funding from UK and European translational research schemes in

order to meet future clinical unmet needs, and carry forward new and innovative ideas.

- For patients in Wales to be consistently offered the opportunity to participate in clinical research and play a greater role in global drug discovery programmes, new technologies and medical devices.
- For NHS R&D to build on existing strengths and consistently deliver commercial research studies in a competitive, global environment.
- For government to work together to promote Wales as a distinctive brand within UK PLC.[1]

Further, since its inception in 2002, the All-Wales Medicines Strategy Group (AWMSG) has forged a strong partnership between NHS Wales and the pharmaceutical industry on the medicines management agenda, and in particular on access to new medicines. In 2017, Health Technology Wales was established to mirror the work of the AWMSG for other health innovations, including devices and diagnostics.

In conclusion

It can be seen that the vibrant Life Sciences industry sector in Wales is well recognised as a strong driver of economic growth, provides highly-skilled employment opportunities and, of vital importance, through the development of innovative medicines and medical technologies, contributes to the delivery of high-quality healthcare.

Recommendation

The people of Wales, community and healthcare professionals, academic groups and the NHS must continue to work together with the Life Science industry in Wales to ensure a prudent agenda for the wellbeing and health for all the people of Wales.

There are good examples of how joint workings can, and have, benefitted the lives of patients and those who care for them in Wales as well as providing economically prudent Healthcare. There are still many medical conditions that could benefit from such partnerships. These should be prioritised and efficient projects created that can deliver benefit in a timely manner.

References

1. http://www.wales.nhs.uk/sites3/documents/952/Industry%20engagement%20
in%20Wales.pdf

12

An overview of global health challenges

Lt General (Ret) Louis Lillywhite CB MBE OStJ

Louis retired as Surgeon General of the UK Armed Forces in 2010. His 42-year career in the Army included medical appointments as a Consultant Occupational Physician, operational deployments, and Command and Staff appointments in the Ministry of Defence and various Army and NATO Headquarters. Since retirement from the Army he has worked as a Senior Research Consultant for the Royal Institute of International Affairs (Chatham House), leading on the relationship between conflict and health. He was also a member of the WHO International Health Regulations Review Committee set up after the 2014 Ebola epidemic. He is a member of the Tribunal Appeal Service for Wales and SW England and a Trustee and past President of the Medical Society of London, President of the Airborne Medical Society, President of his local branch of the Royal British Legion, a Trustee of the Airborne Forces Security Fund, Patron of the Orders of St John Care Trust, Chair of the Welsh Government R&D Division External Strategy Group, and a member of the Royal British Legion Centre for Blast Injury Studies Advisory Board at Imperial College.

This chapter takes a broader look at health, especially as over the last decade it has become a subject that has drawn the attention of world leaders, as exemplified by the involvement of the United Nations in health topics and the initiation of a Global Health Security Track as part of the Munich Security Conference[1] which brings together Heads of State, Foreign and Defence Ministers. Readers may ask why such a chapter be included, to which a quote by Angela Merkel perhaps provides the answer – she said, "Increasingly the health of one person is the health of all. In other words, the effectiveness of the health system in one country has an impact on the health system in other countries." Figure 1 lists the main global health issues, some of which this chapter addresses.

Figure 1 – Current global health issues

Current Global Issues

With a direct impact on the NHS in Wales
        Global healthcare workforce shortage
        Anti-microbial resistance
        Potential pandemic

Other Global Health Issues
        Increased proportion of civilian casualties in conflict
        Attacks on healthcare facilities in conflicts
        Compliance with International Health Regulations
        Impact of counter-terrorist legislation on humanitarian response in some conflict affected areas.

    Medicines: access, affordability, counterfeit and substandard.

From *Combating Infectious Disease to Universal Health Coverage*

Various organisations emerged out of the second World War. The NHS was of course one, but 1948 also saw establishment of the World Health Organization (WHO). Like the NHS, the WHO built on structures that preceded it, namely the Health Organization of the League of Nations (1919) and before that L'Office International d'Hygiene Publique in 1907.[2] Initially, its primary aim was the prevention and control of infectious diseases and in this it has had some notable successes, in particular the elimination of smallpox, the near elimination of polio and the control of the HIV/AIDS global epidemic.

It was not until 1981 that the ambition of the WHO expanded to encompass that which the NHS was formed to do, to provide "Health for All" which was adopted by the 34th World Health Assembly[3] and later articulated by WHO[4] in *Global Strategy for Health for All by the year 2000*. This had its origins in the 1978 Declaration of Alma Ata[5] which noted the "existing gross inequality in the health status of the people particularly between developed and developing countries as well as within countries... is... of common concern to all countries."

By 2000, the WHO "Health for All" had not been achieved and step in the United Nations which in September 2000 committed the world to Millennium Development Goals (MDGs), which were due to be achieved by 2015. Perhaps surprisingly, the concept of "Health for All" did not feature even though universal primary education did. There were however a number of health goals: to reduce child mortality; to improve maternal health; and to combat HIV/AIDS, malaria, and other diseases; and the WHO noted that "the MDGs are inter-dependent; all the MDG influence health, and health influences all the MDGs. For example, better health enables children to learn and adults to earn. Gender equality is essential to the achievement of better health. Reducing poverty, hunger and environmental degradation positively influences, but also depends on, better health."[6] Arguably, the failure to translate "Health for All" into a millennium goal is a demonstration of the limits of both the WHO and individual Health Ministers to influence national and global policies.

In 2015, the eight MDGs were replaced by the 17 UN Sustainable

Development Goals (SDGs) to cover the period until 2030. These goals included many which are highly relevant to health (e.g. number 6, clean water and sanitation and number 10, reduced inequalities). However, SDG 3, 'Good Health and Well-Being' covered the main health goals, comprising 13 specific targets including 3.8: "Achieve universal health coverage, including financial risk protection, access to quality essential healthcare services and access to safe, effective, quality and affordable essential medicines and vaccines for all".[7]

Universal Health Coverage – the world's NHS

Universal Health Coverage (UHC) shares most of the ambitions of those responsible for founding the NHS. It is the replacement for the "Health for All" by the year 2000 which was called for in 1978 and is now a target for 2030. Now, in its 70th year, the WHO is seeking to gain for the global population that which the UK achieved in 1948 on the formation of the NHS, with the WHO "in this 70th anniversary year, calling on world leaders to live up to the pledges they made when they agreed on the Sustainable Development Goals in 2015, and commit to concrete steps to advance #HealthForAll. This means ensuring that everyone, everywhere can access essential quality health services without facing financial hardship."[8] It should be noted that no particular system of healthcare is mandated as individual countries differ in both their philosophies, systems and barriers to healthcare. In many countries, for example, the main barrier to healthcare are the incidental costs (e.g. travel) associated with access to healthcare rather than healthcare itself.

UHC is underpinned by the Tokyo Declaration on Universal Health Coverage[9] which, in essence, replaces the Declaration of Alma Ata. A significant difference is that UHC has the authority provided by a resolution of the United Nations whilst Alma Ata was only underpinned by resolutions of the World Health Assembly. UHC also seems to be gaining traction amongst national politicians, with for example Prime Minister Modi announcing a plan to extend free health care to between 100 and 500 million (press reports differ on the number covered) of India's poorest.

However, there is a major threat to achieving UHC, and indeed to sustaining it in countries such as the UK which have already achieved it. This is the upcoming (some would say current) manpower crisis which is addressed below.

Continuing threats from infectious diseases

Whilst WHO has evolved from an organisation whose almost sole focus was infectious diseases, its role in the prevention, surveillance and control of diseases continues. Infectious disease is common, for example in the week ending 10th May 2018 some 673 new infectious disease alerts were registered.[10] Identifying which of these pose a regional and global threat is the responsibility of WHO and recent outbreaks, such as SARs and H1N1, have been successfully managed.

The system for managing outbreaks requires individual nations to comply with the International Health Regulations 2005.[11] However, in 2014 an outbreak of Ebola, not uncommon in Africa, became out of control and exposed deficiencies in the WHO as well as in international compliance with the International Health Regulations[12] and required international assistance to manage. Indeed, such was the perceived risk to the world that the outbreak was the first disease outbreak to be declared by the UN Security Council as a threat to World Peace[13], resulting in the first UN deployment for the specific purpose of tackling a disease. Indeed, the UN has increasingly become involved in health issues, with it taking a position on attacks on healthcare workers, facilities and patients[14]; the increasing number and proportion of civilian casualties in recent conflicts, where it appears to becoming safer to be a combatant than a civilian[15] whilst the UN Secretary General has even felt the necessity to appoint a high-level panel on healthcare workforce.[16]

A contributing factor to recent major infectious outbreaks not being appropriately managed has been the non-compliance of individual nations with the International Health Regulations, and the recognition of this has led to the introduction of external independent evaluation visits to countries to assess compliance, mainly under the aegis of the Joint External Evaluation (JEE) Alliance which by April 2018 had undertaken 75 inspections.[17] However, such inspections need the agreement of individual States and it remains to be seen the extent to which recommendations following such evaluations are implemented whilst areas of conflict, which arguably pose the greatest risk for the development of a potential pandemic, remain largely outside the global system of surveillance and control. Adding to the risk posed by infectious diseases is the increase in anti-microbial resistance which is assessed in the UK National Risk Register[18] as the top long-term risk facing the UK and indeed is acknowledged by the UN as a global risk.[19]

The (impending) manpower crisis

Extending UHC to the global population requires an expanded and trained workforce. WHO identified[20] a shortfall in 2013 for an additional 17.4 million healthcare professionals (HCPs) with plans only for an additional 3 million by 2030, leaving a deficit of 14.5 million.

However, the more advanced countries aspire to a quality and quantity of healthcare which exceeds that needed for SDGs and WHO estimates[21] that the 31 OECD countries will have an additional shortage by 2030 of 750,000 physicians, 1.1 million nurses and 70,000 Midwives. The US earlier this year produced estimates[22] of its projected deficit and estimates a shortage of between 40,800 and 104,900 physicians by 2030. This shortfall would increase significantly if all US citizens were to enjoy the same level of healthcare as the non-Hispanic white population of USA. The US shortfall included primary care physician shortfall between 7,300 and 43,100 and for 2025 between 7,800 and 32,000, this assuming greater use of nurse practitioners.

Table 1 – Estimates of health worker needs-based shortages (in millions) in countries below the SDG index threshold by region, 2013 and 2030

Region	2013				2030				
	Physicians	Nurses/ midwives	Other cadres	Total	Physicians	Nurses/ midwives	Other cadres	Total	% Change
Africa	0.9	1.8	1.5	4.2	1.1	2.8	2.2	6.1	45%
Americas	0.0	0.5	0.2	0.8	0.1	0.5	0.1	0.6	-17%
Eastern Mediterranean	0.2	0.9	0.6	1.7	0.2	1.2	0.3	1.7	-1%
Europe	0.0	0.1	0.0	0.1	0.0	0.0	0.0	0.1	-33%
South-East Asia	1.3	3.2	2.5	6.9	1.0	1.9	1.9	4.7	-32%
Western Pacific	0.1	2.6	1.1	3.7	0.0	1.2	0.1	1.4	-64%
Grand total	2.6	9.0	5.9	17.4	2.3	7.6	4.6	14.5	-17%

a   Since all values are rounded to the nearest 100 000, totals may not precisely add up.

Source: WHO (2017) Global strategy on human resources for health: Workforce 2030

The global picture is reflected within the UK where in 2015 there was a shortage[23] of 15,000 nurses. The GP figures for 2015[24] showed an estimated decrease of 657 (1.9%) from the 2014 estimated Full Time Equivalent figures, partially offset within primary care by increase of 336 nurses. The NHS Centre for Workforce Planning identifies a major demand-supply imbalance by 2020 under a wide range of scenarios, reaching 190,000 additional clinical posts by 2027.[25]

So, there is a global market place for healthcare workers, and we in the UK are competing with USA and other countries for HCPs from Africa and Asia. Some still think that we can continue to make up any deficit by paying more or recruiting from poorer nations, a policy which has arguably sustained the NHS since its inception and which continues with for example NHS England hoping to cover its increasing shortfall by recruiting from overseas[26] 2,000 doctors over the next three years. However, the second trend will make this more difficult. This is the continuing global economic advances expected over the next decade. Already extreme poverty has been reduced from 44% in 1981 to 11% in 2013 but, more relevant is the expansion in middle classes over next decade which is likely to be the greatest in history, but uneven from only 0.5% per year in OECD countries to 6% per year in emerging economies or, to put it another way, 88% of the next billion people who join the middle classes will be Asian.[27]

This new middle class, mainly Asian, is going to want medical care, especially as Non-Communicable Diseases are increasing, and what is more these increasingly wealthier countries will be able to afford to retain their doctors and nurses instead of exporting them to the UK and other high income countries.

So, the UK has a significant and increasing deficit of HCPs; greater competition for those which are available; and a greater ability by those who currently export healthcare workers to compete for the available HCPs. Some look to prevention as an answer, but whilst strategies to improve the health of the population will undoubtedly improve the quality of life, it is questionable if such strategies will reduce the requirement for healthcare or healthcare workers. Indeed, modelling in the USA on the impact of improved population health is that whilst the physician requirement would reduce in the short term there would be a subsequent increase by the equivalent of an additional 15,000 physicians. After all, everyone must die and the end of life is the period when there is the greatest need for healthcare. The introduction of the NHS was of course also meant to lead to a healthier population which subsequently needed less healthcare and care is needed that this naïve belief is not repeated today! Prevention should of course remain a priority as there are personal, societal and economic benefits to be derived from a fitter and healthier population but we must not look to it to resolve our workforce crisis.

The future – towards different models of healthcare

It is possible that the first 70 years of the NHS will in retrospect be the 'golden years' with Universal Health Coverage provided, but enabled by an internationally recruited workforce. The future is not bright unless we have a fundamental change in how we deliver health care. The impending manpower crisis dwarfs the issues of increased ill health, increased cost of new technology, multi-morbidity and increased expectations of medical care. Tinkering at the edges, such as making medicines cheaper, or some of the innovations we in the Bevan Commission have been supporting is insufficient. Such is the shortfall in manpower that innovations which do not address the manpower shortages will be insufficient.

Over the next 70 years we will need a different model of healthcare which recruits the population as allies and willing partners, recognising their needs but which includes self-care, family care, and care by community. There may be a need to recognise that State cannot provide everything, but where the dividing line lies is an issue for our politicians, as advised and guided by the future managers and workforce of our NHS and social services. A future model is unclear but needs to integrate the care pathway - including primary, secondary and tertiary care - and social care. It must take a "health in all policies approach" and be a model which is based on competence rather than profession and which "task shifts" so that healthcare professions concentrate on that which only they can provide and delegate (with appropriate safeguards). Such a model needs to think beyond current boundaries, be able to mobilise the public in a meaningful way and may well make our craft based professional outlook obsolete. In essence, maintaining the NHS model of care free at the point of delivery will need a revolution in how we use the available workforce.

1948 saw the start of major change in health care provision and its authors faced opposition and entrenched agendas. Their successors in 2018 face no different a situation.

References

1. https://www.securityconference.de/en/activities/health-security-series/ (accessed 10 May 2018)
2. *The Lancet*, Vol 360, October 12, 2002 • www.thelancet.com
3. Resolution WHA34.36
4. WHO Geneva 1981 http://iris.wpro.who.int/bitstream/handle/10665.1/6967/WPR_RC032_GlobalStrategy_1981_en.pdf (accessed 8 May 2018)
5. http://www.euro.who.int/__data/assets/pdf_file/0009/113877/E93944.pdf?ua=1 (accessed 8 May 2018)
6. http://www.who.int/topics/millennium_development_goals/about/en/ (accessed 8 May 2018)
7. http://www.who.int/sdg/targets/en/ (accessed 8 May 2018)
8. http://www.who.int/universal_health_coverage/en/ (accessed 8 May 2018)
9. http://www.who.int/universal_health_coverage/tokyo-decleration-uhc.pdf?ua=1
10. www.healthmap.org/en/ (accessed 10 May 2018)
11. *International Health Regulations 2005 3rd Edition* see www.who.int/ihr/publications/9789241580496/en/ (accessed 8 May 2018)
12. *The (2016) Review Committee on the Role of the International Health Regulations (2005) in the Ebola Outbreak and Response* - http://www.who.int/ihr/review-committee-2016/en/ (accessed 8 May 2018)
13. UN Security Council Resolution 2177 (2014) of 18 Sep 2014 – text at http://www.ifrc.org/docs/IDRL/UN%20SC%20Res.pdf (accessed 8 May 2018)
14. UN Security Council Resolution 2286: https://www.un.org/press/en/2016/sc12347.doc.htm (accessed 8 May 2018)
15. Guha-Sapir et al; *Patterns of civilian and child deaths due to war-related violence in Syria: a comparative analysis from the Violation Documentation Center dataset, 2011–16; Lancet Global Health DOI*: https://doi.org/10.1016/S2214-109X(17)30469-2
16. United Nations Secretary - General High-Level Commission on Health Employment and Economic Growth established 20 Sep 2016 - http://www.oecd.org/els/health-systems/unsg-high-level-commission-on-health-employment-and-economic-growth.htm (accessed 8 May 2018)
17. See https://www.jeealliance.org/ (accessed 10 May 2018)
18. National Risk Register of Civil Emergencies – 2017 Edition Cabinet Office
19. http://www.who.int/en/news-room/detail/21-09-2016-at-un-global-leaders-commit-to-act-on-antimicrobial-resistance (accessed 10 May 2018)
20. http://who.int/hrh/resources/global_strategy_workforce2030_14_print.pdf?ua=1 Table A1.3
21. Ibid pp 44-45

22. https://aamc-black.global.ssl.fastly.net/production/media/filer_public/c9/db/c9dbe9de-aabf-457f-aee7-1d3d554ff281/aamc_projections_update_2017_final_-_june_12.pdf
23. https://improvement.nhs.uk/uploads/documents/Clinical_workforce_report.pdf
24. http://content.digital.nhs.uk/catalogue/PUB20503/nhs-staf-2005-2015-gene-prac-rep.pdf
25. Public Health England; *Facing the Facts, Shaping the Future: A draft health and care workforce strategy for England to 2027*
26. https://www.england.nhs.uk/gp/gpfv/workforce/building-the-general-practice-workforce/international-gp-recruitment/
27. https://www.brookings.edu/wp-content/uploads/2017/02/global_20170228_global-middle-class.pdf

13

Building community capacity and resilience - engaging and empowering people and communities

Fran Targett OBE

Fran has been associated with Citizens Advice since 1978, when she started as a volunteer adviser, and was appointed Director of Citizens Advice Cymru in 2000, responsible for Citizens Advice services across Wales. She sits on the Wales Council for Voluntary Action Board, represents the Advice and Advocacy sector on the Third Sector Partnership Council and chairs the Wales Independent Advice Providers Forum and is currently a member of the Welsh Government's National Advice Network.

It is important to consider the contribution from individuals, communities and the third sector in delivering a truly prudent approach to health and social care. The prudent principles explicitly state that it is essential to achieve health and wellbeing with the public, patients and professionals as equal partners through co-production. It is important to unpick what this will mean for people as well as for health and care professionals. This means consideration of the ethos of reciprocity, the value of volunteering and the added value of the third sector leading to how joint ownership of health and wellbeing can be achieved.

In the Bevan Commission paper, *Redrawing the relationship between the citizen and the state* (Bevan Commission, February 2016) the relationship was characterised as potentially being on a continuum between passivity and co-production.

Figure 1 - Power / Impact Continuum

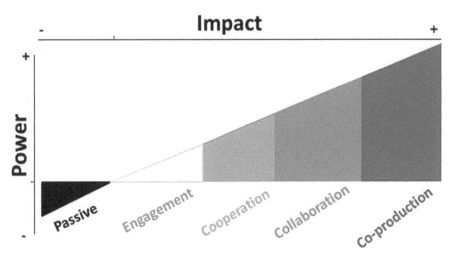

In addition, a useful consideration would be between the concepts of reciprocity and altruism. The ethos of reciprocity implies that people operate against the practice of giving and receiving, it could be argued that this is as simple as people paying through their national insurance and taxes to receive health and social care from the state. In addition, some see health and social care as having an element of altruism where people who cannot afford to pay their contribution continue to receive the services according to need, arguably meeting the prudent principle to care for those with the greatest health need first, making most effective use of all skills and resources.

However, reciprocity can be interpreted much more widely, the Cambridge English Dictionary defines it as a reciprocal action or arrangement involves two people or groups of people who behave in the same way or agree to help each other and give each other advantages. In this context, it is important to understand a complex relationship between people and their own health. Moving to a place where as well as 'giving' through taxes people see themselves as directly responsible for their personal contribution to their own and their family's health and care. In the Bevan paper, *Redrawing the relationship between the citizen and the state* (Bevan Commission, February 2016) it was made clear that the Well-being of Future Generations (Wales) Bill (Welsh Government, 2015) recognises that to give future generations a good quality of life we must work together to tackle the challenges of today and tomorrow to improve the social, economic, environmental and cultural wellbeing of Wales. We therefore need a real commitment to real change in the relationship between citizens and the state. This could go beyond the 'simple' co-production approach to each individual's health and care to an attitude of a membership style relationship between people and the health care system and professionals, where the relationship is equalised and individuals can expect specific services and responses and the state also can expect that individuals and groups help them to achieve health and wellbeing.

It is important that we recognise the parts of civic society which are outside the health and care systems but which improve people's health and to actively encourage these to continue is vital. Research has shown that, in addition to providing positive actions and activities for society, volunteering is good for your health and wellbeing. It will be important to continue to encourage volunteering opportunities to achieve improved and prudent health outcomes. The report commissioned by Volunteering England in 2008 and carried out by the University of Wales Lampeter, *Volunteering and Health: What Impact Does It Really Have?* concluded that[1]: in the health impact for volunteers, volunteering was shown to decrease mortality and to improve self-rated health, mental health, life satisfaction, the ability to carry out activities of daily living without functional impairment, social support and interaction, healthy behaviours and the ability to cope with one's own illness.

In addition, the article Association of volunteering with mental wellbeing: a life-course analysis of a national population-based longitudinal study in the UK[2], published in the BMJ concluded:

> *Previous studies have reported better mental well-being using the GHQ among those involved in volunteering activities. Our study indicates that the relationship between volunteering and mental well-being varies across the life course, which suggests that volunteering may be more strongly associated with mental well-being at some points of the life course than others. There is no clear evidence that volunteering was positively associated with mental health during early adulthood to mid-adulthood. Rather, the positive association began to become apparent after around 40 years and continued up to old age. Those who never volunteered seemed to have lower levels of mental well-being starting around midlife and continuing in old age compared to those involved in volunteering. These associations between mental well-being and volunteering are robust to a range of potential confounders, which are used in adjusting the models.*

Given the specific concerns about increased demand for health and care services given the aging nature of our population it will be very important for the future wellbeing for older people this research that these volunteering opportunities are encouraged.

The WCVA reports that there are over 33,000 voluntary, community and not-for-profit organisations in Wales and the Wales Omnibus survey 2014/15 estimated that 938,175 people volunteer with an organisation in Wales. WCVA's database indicates that in the region of 12% of these organisations are working directly in the health and social care sector and the Volunteering in Wales 2015 Report on two Omnibus surveys March 2014 and 2015[3] reports that 16.4% of the volunteering population (6.1% of the total adult population) of Wales provide volunteer support for organisations engaged around health, disability and social welfare. This shows that there is already a substantial engagement and commitment from the third sector. Given that this sector is predominantly charitable, these organisations operate within the charitable purpose for the public benefit and that a large proportion of them operate specifically for the prevention or relief of poverty, the advancement of health or the saving of lives and the relief of those in need, by reason of youth, age, ill-health, disability, financial hardship or other disadvantage the overall principles of prudence have a very good chance of being absolutely embedded in the sector's approach.

Some of the sector working within health and social care deliver public funded services alongside their wider charitable approach which brings added value and some deliver services and influence which is in addition to public funded provision through their alternative funding activities. It will be essential in delivering a wider prudent health and care system to harness and encourage the input of the third sector and to adopt its ethos relating to public benefit across other partners. Finding a way to bring the wider public service (rather than public sector) together is vital to ensuring the best outcomes for the people of Wales.

The conclusion that, in addition to those holding statutory responsibility for health and social care, there needs to be encouragement and recognition of the prudent contribution from others in communities, including the wider public sector, community groups and the wider third sector. It will be vital to promote the view that health and wellbeing is jointly owned by individuals and communities. Educating individuals through public health methodologies is important but more importantly a complete mind-set change for joint ownership will need changes across the board.

Alongside the need for major cultural change within the health and social care sectors themselves there is a need for a shift to recognise the value of services which are not apparently directly health related. Increasing understanding of the value to health and wellbeing is characterised by the move towards valuing social prescribing by primary health care providers.

Evidence is growing about the health benefits, particularly for people with long term health conditions, of referrals and joint working across a range of service providers.[4] Current austerity is leaving some service delivery which has been shown to be valuable to health and wellbeing has become more vulnerable to severe and sometimes final cuts and the lack of work to integrate the wider impacts into any changes across the sector. Some of the areas of current concern are the loss of activity and leisure facilities in communities at the time when the health sector is encouraging increased activity as an important element in the treatment of health conditions related to obesity including diabetes[5] but also in mental health[6] and work-related conditions.[7] The links between advice, particularly on debt and income maximisation on mental health are clearly articulated in literature review from the Royal College of Psychiatrists in Debt and mental health, *What do we know? What should we do?*[8] that concludes:

> *A renewed emphasis on co-ordinated 'debt care pathways' between local health and advice services – that is, the routes by which individuals with debt and mental health problems gain access to the support they need – may be key.*

In conclusion, the approach that 'We're all in this together' means that individuals, communities, organisations as well as the health and care providers will need to work closely together to understand the whole system which impacts on people's wellbeing and health. A realistic approach which ceases to blame the health and care sector for our increasingly unrealistic demands as a society but also engages in jointly owned solutions where everyone takes personal as well as organisational responsibility, that the relationship is one of joint ownership and reciprocity.

Whilst we may not have all the answers as to how best to achieve this, there is a need to start somewhere, stimulating people in conversations around this and in finding new ideas and solutions with them, sharing and learning from each other along the way. Doing so will help not only develop better services, it will also help develop a more trusting and rebalanced relationship with the very people we are trying to help.

The conclusion of the Bevan Commission paper remains the essential first steps in achieving this the new relationship required.

1. Co-production principles are embedded into every aspect of the work of health and social care at national and local levels as a fundamental prerequisite of all working practices, aligning resources, targets and incentives accordingly.

2. Training and support for health and care professionals at all levels will need to be revised to support the change of emphasis and shift of power. Professional bodies, training and education organisations, audit and inspection bodies will all need to reflect this change. We recommend that all practitioners in health and social care use the phrase 'what can we do together' in place of 'what can I do for you?'

3. A national conversation and campaign are initiated to ensure everyone understands and are able to fully participate, drawing from evidence in health literacy and behaviour change.

4. Key organisations in Wales such as: Community Health Councils; Wales Audit Office; Healthcare Inspectorate Wales; Care and Social Services Inspectorate Wales; and professional representative bodies should all take full account of their role and responsibility in redrawing the relationship between the citizen and the state.

References

1. https://www.scribd.com/document/352350841/Volunteering-and-Health-What-impact-does-it-really-have
2. http://bmjopen.bmj.com/content/6/8/e011327 2016
3. https://www.wcva.org.uk/media/4576349/final_volunteering_in_wales_2015_-_english_july_2016.pdf
4. http://www.primarycareone.wales.nhs.uk/sitesplus/documents/1191/Social%20prescribing%20inclusions%20for%20evidence%20map.pdf
5. http://eprints.gla.ac.uk/96486/
6. https://www.cambridge.org/core/journals/public-health-nutrition/article/influence-of-physical-activity-on-mental-wellbeing/3C363AEECE5C8CAC490A585BA29E6BF8
7. http://bjsm.bmj.com/content/43/1/47.short
8. https://www.rcpsych.ac.uk/pdf/Debt%20and%20mental%20health%20(lit%20review%20-%2009_10_18).pdf

Bevan Commission (2016). *Redrawing the relationship between the citizen and the state*

Welsh Government (2015). Well-being of Future Generations (Wales) Act. Available at: http://gov.wales/docs/dsjlg/publications/150623-guide-to-the-fg-act-en.pdf

14

Engaging the wisdom and resources of people and patients in their health, care and wellbeing

Mary Cowern

Mary has spent the last 20 years working in a needs-led environment within the third sector. She currently holds a senior leadership post in Arthritis Care as Wales Director, ensuring the strategic development and funding of the charities operational services in Wales. As well as leading on the Nation's policy and public affairs agenda, she also provides a devolved perspective on the charity's Senior Management Team and has the UK oversight of Arthritis Care's Living Well with Arthritis Services. She is a patient partner with OMERACT (linked to the Cochrane Collaboration Musculoskeletal Review Group) and is Chair of the Long Term Conditions Alliance Cymru, participates in a number of Welsh Government working groups, task groups and boards and is a member of the Welsh Arthritis Research Network (WARN).

The rhetoric of co-production, citizen involvement and the aspiration to give people more control over their own health and wellbeing is not a new one. We know that the public, patients and their careers need to be in the driving seat, ensuring care and support is built around what matters to them most. However, despite being enshrined in Welsh policy we are still a long way from establishing co-production and self-care as the everyday norm for our citizens. With increasing demands and dwindling resources, providing healthcare in the way that we have done is no longer an option. Our citizens must take responsibility for their health and wellbeing if we are to ensure our NHS is fit for the future. But how do we engage the wisdom and resources of people and patients in their health, care and wellbeing – how do we bridge that gap from rhetoric to reality?

Too often health is seen as someone else's problem – the chain smoking, overweight 50-year-old who relies on blood pressure medication, who can't exercise because their "joints are too bad", who's only health worry when visiting their GP is questioning why they've been waiting so long for a hip replacement. We have fallen into a society which has become medicalised within a predominantly biomedical model of care. Since the inception of the NHS the public have adopted the notion of 'doctor knows best', 'I am ill and my doctor will make me better'. Similarly, for too long patients have been passive recipients of care, controversially derived from patients defining professionals by the knowledge and power they hold. Attitudes are changing and with our growing information explosion and advances in technology, health knowledge is now open to everyone. However, barriers are still evident, and attitudes are not changing as fast as our technology is evolving.

A recent survey by the Kings Fund (2017) found that two-thirds of the public (65 per cent) agree that keeping healthy is primarily the responsibility of the individual, while just 7 per cent put this responsibility on the NHS. Therefore, if acceptance is there, the question arises as to whether it is an issue of motivation, capacity or both which prevents many of our patients and public taking charge of their own health and wellbeing?

For some people, using health services responsibly may offer little personal benefit i.e. the cost of treating a minor ailment via over the counter treatments may seem too costly. However, 'irresponsible' use may be rewarded with the promise of free and prompt treatment e.g. in the case of choosing to attend an A&E department with a minor problem and being treated 'for free'. Lower income families may have concerns over the cost of healthier food and are at odds with quality vs quantity. Inexpensive junk food can often seem more appealing when budgets are tight, leading to unhealthy dietary habits and subsequent health problems.

We are constantly presented with advice to exercise more, eat healthily, drink less or read in the media how something is good for you one day and bad the next. With so many mixed messages it's no wonder the public become confused. Misinformation or lack of knowledge and education can lead people to miss out on making the right choices when it comes to wellbeing. To make good choices, individuals need to understand the consequences and take responsibility for them. Throw in the intricacies and complexities of individuals who experience low health literacy and we enter a whole different ball game. The practical challenge is how can we promote a culture of choice that involves responsible, informed and supported decision-making that all can take part in regardless of their level of knowledge, experience or health literacy?

On an average day in Wales over 46,000 people contact their GP, nearly 2,750 people attend an Emergency Department and more than 1,250 calls are made to the Welsh Ambulance Service (Welsh NHS Confederation, 2018). In 2002, Wanless outlined a vison for "tomorrow's patient" who would be better informed, more empowered and engaged in their wellbeing yet demand on our NHS still remains high. We know patients want to be more involved in their care. On a typical day NHS Direct Wales receives over 800 calls and over 9,000 website visits (Welsh NHS Confederation, 2018), suggesting that on balance citizens in Wales are making choices and decisions every day about how to manage their health. We also know that on average people living with long term health conditions spend just 3 hours a year with health professionals. The remaining 8,757 hours in a year are spent managing their own condition (www.Self-ManagementUK.org). Evidently not all our citizens are passive recipients of care thus we need to better understand what drives and empowers individuals to take action when others do not.

There is increasingly strong evidence that patients who understand and manage their condition and who are involved in decisions about their care have better outcomes. An evidence review by the Health Foundation (De Silva, 2011) suggests that supporting people to look after themselves can improve their motivation, the extent to which they eat well and exercise, improve their symptoms and clinical outcomes and can even change how they use health services which echoes my own personal experience. Having lived with rheumatoid arthritis for over 30 years I have first-hand experience of moving from being a passive recipient of care to an empowered individual in charge of my own health. The journey to take control over my wellbeing certainly wasn't easy, and I needed motivation and support to get me there. My diagnosis was a complete shock. I was told that by the time I was 30 I would be in a wheelchair, there was no cure and I'd just have to live with it. Not the best thing to be told when you are only 20 and have your whole life ahead of you! Due to my lack of understanding of my condition and the way my diagnosis was presented to me I went into 'sick' mode. I found myself faced with a daunting array of treatments and services, which I knew nothing about. I'd suddenly gone from being independent and lively to someone friends and family felt sorry for. I was in constant pain, becoming increasing immobile and unsurprisingly depression was setting in. Trying to merely function each day was exhausting. I felt that I'd lost control, not only of my health but also of my life too.

My turning point came when I was able to take ownership of my condition and start regaining my independence. In everyday life we utilise numerous skills to enable us to function such as problem solving, planning, and decision-making. We use most of these skills as a matter of course, however I found when I was faced with such a life changing situation my 'rational' thinking went out the window. I had so many things that I had to deal with such as isolation, pain, diminishing independence, capacity to work and look after my family, financial and practical worries. I didn't just need medical treatment I need extra support to help put things into perspective.

My motivation to take responsibility for my health was when I met others who truly understood, it was about building my confidence back and my capacity to take charge. I began to break out of the 'sick mode' I'd fallen into. I'd made the decision that this wasn't going to beat me – if others could do it so could I. The way you think about your condition certainly influences how you deal with it. I started to look at what I could do rather than what I couldn't. Talking to others who had lived with the condition made me realise there were things I could do it wasn't the end of the world. I attended a self-management course and learnt how to set goals for myself, how to become better informed about my condition and communicate effectively with my health care team and family. I learnt how to practice self-care principles such as pacing myself, managing my condition by healthy eating, practicing relaxation techniques and safe exercise. I now practice self-care principles every day without even thinking about it. I gained the confidence to have constructive, informed dialogues with my healthcare team. We became a partnership, myself and my healthcare team working towards the same goal. We made decisions together – I was in charge and our shared decision making made a marked difference my treatment outcomes.

Nevertheless, telling someone to practice self-care is not enough - you need to be motivated or your journey will fail. However, lack of confidence, self-esteem and encouragement create barriers to motivation. I was lucky, I'm a pretty resilient person and found the motivation and confidence to embark on my journey, however many aren't as fortunate and need extra support to achieve this. If we are to successfully create a culture where people practice self-care as a norm we must understand what will help people more effectively manage their own health and wellbeing from their personal perspective and not from a condition perspective. For me it was creating behaviour change via different approaches, but it started with peer support and information. The power of learning from your peers cannot be underestimated. Having the right information, pitched at the right level and delivered in the right context is incredibly empowering, all of which is fundamental to co-production and prudent health care.

We shouldn't be fooled into thinking that merely giving information or referring someone onto a self-management workshop is enough either. It is unlikely that one off interventions will make a significant impact, so we must understand the journeys individuals will need to take. The Health Foundation (De Silva, 2011) illustrates the differing typologies and positions of self-management support along a continuum depicted in Figure 1.

Figure 1 – Continuum strategies to support self-management

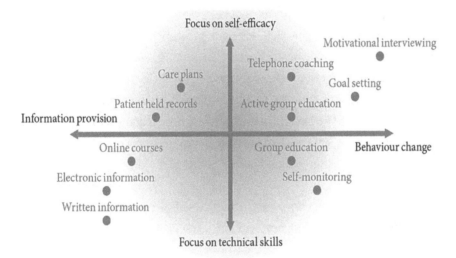

A one size approach will not fit all – patients and the public are all individual, with different needs and values. Most people cope and manage minor illnesses without seeking professional help because they know what to do and are confident in taking action. However, for some in society that's not the case.

It is evident that even when people know what the 'healthy' and right thing to do is, and have the desire to act, they often encounter barriers to see their intentions through. Awareness and intention aren't always enough – we need to find ways of helping people change their behaviour. The challenge is finding the most effective ways of supporting, enabling and sustaining change. We need to exploit the potential of our peers – connecting with people who we see as being like us can have a strong influence on behaviour and in turn our wellbeing.

We must invest time and energy to change thinking. It might feel quicker for a health professional to merely tell individuals to change habits or advise people on lifestyle changes, but that just increases dependency on the professional and the system. More importantly, it misses out on the opportunity to encourage citizens to come up with ideas and solutions themselves – a far more empowering and sustainable solution. Health care professionals often do not receive any formal training in enabling patients and carers to manage their own health. We need to ensure health professionals truly understand the value of such an approach and are given the skills, tools and confidence to empower patients and the public to be active and equal partners in their care.

Our ambition for sustainable prudent healthcare in Wales, where everyone is involved in and has responsibility for addressing the challenges ahead, can only happen if there is a will and desire to do things differently. We as citizens, patients, public and professionals must be bold, we must think differently and champion the possible. We need to lead by example, show how empowering it is to take charge of our own health and wellbeing – we need to motivate, enable and support desires into actions and influence culture and behaviour change. Only then will cultures shift from passive recipients of care to empowered individuals taking charge of their health and wellbeing. We need to secure a platform for future generations to think and act differently. Our future model must provide fundamental elements which encourage, promote and support the ability of the citizen to maintain health, adapt to challenges and to practice self-care if we are to realise our aspirations of forming a new relationship between our citizens and our services.

References

de Silva, D. (2011). *Helping people help themselves.* The Health Foundation. Available online at: www.health.org.uk/publications/evidence-helping-people-help-themselves

Kings Fund. (2017). *What does the public think about the NHS?* Available online at: https://www.kingsfund.org.uk/publications/what-does-public-think-about-nhs

Wanless, D. (2002). *Securing our Future Health: Taking a Long-Term View* http://si.easp.es/derechosciudadania/wp-content/uploads/2009/10/4.Informe-Wanless.pdf

Welsh NHS Confederation. (2018). *On an average day in NHS Wales* – Welsh. http://www.nhsconfed.org/resources/2018/02/on-an-average-day-in-nhs-wales-welsh

15

The community infrastructure – a crucial component of community health

Dr Helen Paterson

Helen is the Chief Executive at Walsall Council and has previously held a number of senior local authority posts including Chief Executive, Strategic Director for Transformation, and Executive Director of Children's Services. Helen is a JP; a member of a wide range of ministerial and national groups; and Visiting Professor at Glyndwr University.

What if our current NHS 'medical' model (which, in the simplest of terms, focusses on illness and getting people well again) evolved into an NHS 'social' model which focused on wellbeing, healthy lifestyles and diet, and purposeful quality living? A model in which individuals and communities were more responsible for their own wellbeing and health outcomes? In essence, one in which local people, communities and groups lead in their own localities to determine the best outcomes for themselves and received appropriate support to achieve these.

I believe that this may be possible without the need for massive structural change or a huge financial intervention. What is needed is a mind-set which moves away from the almost learned 'helplessness and dependency', to one where people are enabled to take control of their own wellbeing and health in their own localities. The infrastructure necessary to achieve this comprises of much more than that directly related to health and illness or medicines and interventions.

Some aspects of this change from a medical to a social model would, undoubtedly, require expenditure. It may, for example, include the need for better quality housing or more housing provision which is better designed and more readily available to meet a wider range of social and medical needs. But community infrastructure, in its widest sense can often be modified without substantial initial expenditure and, after some 'pump-priming' could indeed be more financially efficient. Could, for example, more 'purposeful living' be brought about by increasing paid employment opportunities? This could be achieved perhaps by better tackling prejudice that may prevent certain groups benefitting from the current growth in employment and by addressing skills shortages in certain sectors of the economy.

Could there be a more systematic approach to enable volunteering within communities? We could create places that enable people to share their leisure time and creativity. This model is underpinned by design principles that start with the needs of individuals in their localities and communities and so requires a community infrastructure which meets need on a more human scale than that which underpins much existing practice.

Currently I believe we have created, with the best of initial intentions, a NHS that people have become dependent upon to the extent that 'the system' has taken away much of the need to be mindful and aware of the responsibility for one's own wellbeing. This 'helplessness' then perpetuates itself by creating more and more demand to fulfil the perceived needs expressed in medical terms. So, then a vicious circle develops of reinforcing the 'way the system' works and perhaps, more worryingly, a vicious circle of 'getting around the system'.

An elderly lady phones a local authority switchboard a dozen times a day just so that she has someone to talk to. A middle-aged man calls 999 for an ambulance several times a day because he knows someone will come and he will have company. These two examples are not uncommon. They are not about illness or health care or interventions. They are about loneliness and isolation and a desire for human contact and discourse. They are about a lack of access to regular public transport and a lack of places to meet. Maybe also (after a prolonged period of behaving this way) there is less desire to get out and about because the people concerned have found a way to meet their perceived needs.

Some people dial 999 because they need paracetamol (they really do) or because they have run out of their prescription medicine or their pizza takeaway delivery is late. To most people these examples may beggar belief, but they have all happened. These 999 callers simply did not think that, if paracetamol or pizza is what they needed, they could source it themselves at a local chemist or a supermarket.

Where local authorities provide night shelters for the homeless, the main issues that present themselves are often not those concerned with the availability of suitable accommodation (such as the ability to find work with no fixed address). Rather, they relate to mental health, to drug and alcohol addiction and to a lack of purposeful activity to fill the long hours before the shelter opens again for the night. Within one such shelter in the West Midlands in 2017, of the 31 regular visitors 12 were quickly helped into appropriate accommodation whilst others were helped into employment and training and others were assisted on mental health supported programmes. The broader issue of course was why was there a need for the night shelter in the first place?

Is the key to addressing some of these issues people who can work together in local communities? Service professionals and volunteers and service users all coming together to design what their community needs? Working bottom up? Design based on what local people would like to see happening? Or organisations deciding what they think people need, commissioning activities to those needs and expecting people to 'tailor themselves' to the services available?

An elderly lady I know was speaking to her community advocate (who worked for the local authority with a role as local 'connector' of people and activities) talking about her love of playing the game Scrabble and how she had no one to play with. Through the library and local shop (with her community advocate's support) she found several people in her community, in the streets just by her, that love Scrabble. They have now set up a weekly Scrabble Club and take it in turns each week to host the club at each other's homes. Was there a massive service restructure necessary or a huge amount of money invested? No. There was a person acting as a 'connector' of like-minded people who now have a new activity, company and purpose in their lives. A new group of Scrabblers (or whatever the collective noun is for those who play Scrabble), has been established in a community by the community. It is possible that this development has prevented that lady from becoming the 999 caller who simply has not had anyone to talk to for days or even weeks. This small example is scalable.

All over the country local authorities with locality-based services are joining with other organisations and groups, both from the statutory, third and faith sectors (which also provide locality based services) to work with individuals and communities to help redesign services to meet local needs. Local authorities are supporting community groups to work jointly through short term loans and grants. Community-funded, voluntary sector organisations are guiding local groups to enable them to access a range of other funding sources like charities and the lottery.

In jargon terms, communities are building their 'social capital'. Like-minded folk are 'time banking' - that is, banking their time as a 'currency' to share between their communities for gardening, dog walking, babysitting, theatre groups and book clubs. In a small Welsh village of just 75 houses and no public transport or public amenities (other than a post box and a notice board) local people have formed a charity, bought a disused old hut and set up a community hall with a book club, fitness classes, quiz nights and jigsaw parties. The community coming together to take responsibility themselves for their own wellbeing activities, encouraging social cohesion and intergenerational activities and having fun. Locally together, taking social responsibility.

In a prudent approach the examples I have given help to build individual and community wellbeing through developing strong communities.

The challenge is to address the constantly growing demand for services and the expectation that these will also be of greater quality. This in turn can, if not tackled correctly, perpetuate a non-prudent approach and reinforce a lack of personal responsibility and accountability. This is exacerbated by our ageing population, skills shortages and major fiscal challenges, alongside the need to safeguard and protect individuals through greater regulation.

The response must be to determine how we can best evolve a social model to the provision of services generally and, in particular, in the NHS. How do we move from endless crisis, such as the annual winter pressures upon accident and emergency services? This evolution will require organisational goals to be adjusted to strive for place-based, co-designed and delivered sets of integrated, localised services, in which we work with local communities and encourage personal responsibility and so better meet the needs of the individuals within these communities.

The starting point, therefore, may be the development of common shared population-based outcomes, across organisations and sectors.

Call to action

My call to action:

- Stop thinking first of services and service delivery. Instead think of places and people. Think of how their needs (such as transport, housing, jobs, health, social and leisure) interrelate. Then design services and service delivery mechanisms around these.

- Stand in the shoes of the individual. Ask what sense an individual can make of all the organisations, activities and pathways for service delivery in their locality. Ask whether individuals have to 'tailor themselves' to fit what is available? Establish common shared population outcomes, agreed by local people as relevant to their lives and their needs.

- Do not commission and provide services through inertia because they have always been provided. Ending any service will inevitably face some public opposition. Have the courage to ask whether some can be decommissioned because others will meet needs more effectively. This in turn will increase efficiency. Design these new services locally, and deliver locally whenever possible, through shared activity and co-location. And put people first by ending the 'turf wars' that inhibit the development of shared joint budgets and preciousness about who can do what.

I believe this call-to-arms can create a sustainable community infrastructure in which individuals take responsibility for their own wellbeing and health outcomes. Will you join me?

16

Education, skills and training for sustainable health and care within Wales

Professor Hywel Thomas CBE

Hywel is ProVice-Chancellor, Research, Innovation and Engagement at Cardiff University. In this role he is responsible for the University's research activities and its engagement with innovation, including commercialisation and the broader economic impact of the University.

Professor Thomas is also a Professor of Civil Engineering, Director of the Geoenvironmental Research Centre (GRC) and a UNESCO Professor in the Development of a Sustainable Geoenvironment.

Helen Howson

Helen is the Director of the Bevan Commission and the Bevan Commission Academy. She has played a lead role in its establishment and in the development of Prudent Healthcare and the Bevan Innovators and Bevan Innovation Hub programmes. She was previously a Public Health Consultant with Public Health Wales which involved leading a major ministerial review of health improvement interventions across Wales and wider service improvement. Prior to this Helen held a number of senior positions within Welsh Government Health Policy and Strategy over a 12-year period, latterly heading up the Primary and Community Health Strategy Unit.

Where are we now? What skills do we have?

Wales can be rightly proud of its current position in relation to the education, skills and training agenda for sustainable health and care. Our 'Education, Skills and Training' sector is of a high international standard, recognised as such worldwide. The sector is both comprehensive and diverse, from nursery education through to further and higher education and onto lifelong learning.

The range of skills deployed in these organisations is enormous, including for example medical, dental, nursing, therapists, scientists, engineers, planners and catering staff. As has been stated many times by numerous commentators, the dedication and professionalism of the health and care work force is on display for all to see, every hour of the day, every day of the week and every week of the year.

The health and care sector employs a very large number of people. The current NHS workforce in Wales is made up of approximately 89,000 people (Figure 1). This is around 4.5% of the 16-64 age group in Wales. Social Care Wales (2017) publishes workforce data on Social Workers in Wales which highlights the 3,900 registered social workers employed in local authorities at the end of March 2016. In relation to the Volunteer Sector, it is estimated that there are over 33,000 third sector organisations working in Wales. Within these there are 938,000 volunteers. Carers Wales (2018) report that over 380,000 people provide unpaid care for disabled, seriously ill or older loved one in Wales.

Figure 1: Employed[a] NHS Wales staff in Wales September 2016[b]

The total number (FTE[c]) of directly employed NHS staff	76,288
Medical & dental staff	6,233
Hospital medical and dental consultants	2,369
Nursing, midwifery and health visiting staff	29,388
Scientific, therapeutic & technical staff	12,429
Administration & estates staff	16,570
Other staff (inc. healthcare assistants, support staff and ambulance staff)	11,669

Note:

    a)   This data is produced from the Electronic Staff Record (ESR) and as such does not include GPs or Dentists who work as independent contractors, or temporary/agency staff. https://statswales.wales.gov.uk/Catalogue/Health-and-Social-Care/NHS-Staff

    b)   Most up to date available is for 30th September 2016. The data for 2017 is expected to be published in March 2018 http://gov.wales/docs/statistics/ 2017/170329-staff-directly-employed-nhs-30-september-2016-en.pdf

    c)   Full-time equivalent (FTE) numbers are calculated by dividing the number of hours staff in a grade are contracted to work by the standard hours for that grade. In this way, part-time staff are converted into an equivalent number of full-time staff. Over time, FTE is the most appropriate measure of staff resource to use and is used in official statistical releases.

In Wales, we need to look ahead, to build on this excellence and attempt to comment on the various aspects needed to change to "future proof" the system. One of the challenges that will need to be overcome is the current inability to recruit skilled individuals to meet needs, based upon our current model of healthcare.

What will we need for the future?

To change the way the future health and social care workforce is planned and delivered will require a change in culture and ethos consistent with a prudent model of health as outlined by the Bevan Commission (2017). The Well-Being of Future Generations Act (2015) also speaks to this topic and it is imperative that plans for the future provide an important foundation stone for the delivery of the requirements of the Act.

In Wales a new body, Health Education and Improvement Wales (HEIW), has been created[1] to combine the functions undertaken by the Wales Deanery, the Welsh Centre for Postgraduate Pharmacy Education (WCPPE) and the Workforce, Education and Development Services (WEDS) Team within NHS Shared Services. HEIW aim to deliver a single body to support the development of the health workforce in Wales, including education and training, planning, leadership, careers, improvement and widening access. As such HEIW will have a central and leading role to play in achieving this and many other aspects within this paper.

Documentation produced by the HEART (2017) initiative: the Health Enterprise Alliance for Regional Transformation, *A Strategic Blueprint for the Cardiff and Vale Health and Care System* presents the following analysis:

- *Our population is growing... particularly those who currently have a greater dependency on public services... and those with multiple long term conditions.*
- *The burden of disease will increase if nothing changes.*
- *Our public services are already struggling operationally to keep pace with demand.*
- *For our population, we are not realising the benefits of health and care innovation.*
- *We owe it to those we serve, and to those we lead, to change the game, to do for health and wellbeing what Apple did for consumer technology.*

What needs to change?

The development of an education, skills and learning approach that is compatible with the principles of Prudent Health Care (Bevan Commission, 2015) is a priority. As citizens of our nation, we will need to become more mindful of our own responsibilities for our own health and wellbeing. Our education system will need to prepare us for this world.

The future for our society is increasingly a digital future. Future education, skills and training needs will need to accommodate these advances. As we all know, these are rapidly evolving fields where the pace of change can be astonishing, exciting and frightening, all at the same time. We are unlikely to have learnt all our lifetime skills during our formal early years of education, so lifelong learning will be a must. Just as for other sectors, it is also unlikely that our current models of education, skills and learning will all remain fit for purpose as this digital world evolves.

Advances in the impact of science and technology on the Health and Care sector will also continue to need to be addressed. The education, skills and learning agenda will need to accommodate future changes on this front, all of which are also developing at a pace.

We will want our people to be self-sufficient, resilient, flexible, confident, motivated and dynamic. We need to develop the kind of system that will help us achieve this goal. We also need to ensure that they have employment that will encourage them to live and work in Wales.

Building upon what we already have

There are a number of important components already in place, as the foundation stones for the future. Examining these across the educational range, starting with the youngest we have in nursery education, the key requirement is to raise young children's overall awareness of being healthy. Good habits learnt at a young age will then hopefully lead to good health and wellbeing behaviour as adults, where they take responsibility for their own health. The factors of importance include an appreciation of eating well, eating healthy food, knowing where food comes from and the importance of exercise.

For families with children under 4 years of age living in disadvantaged areas of Wales, the Flying Start programme is an important and valuable foundation stone. All aspects of the programme are of potential value, namely: free quality, part-time childcare for 2-3 year olds; an enhanced health visiting service; access to parenting programmes; and speech, language and communication.

The Donaldson (2015) Report, *An Independent Review of Curriculum and Assessment Arrangements in Wales*, is another key development. The

Review developed 'curriculum purposes' to encapsulate a vision of the well-educated learner, completing their statutory education in Wales. These 'purposes' are that all our children / young people will be:

- ambitious, capable learners, ready to learn throughout their lives;
- enterprising, creative contributors, ready to play a full part in life and work;
- ethical, informed citizens of Wales and the world; and
- healthy, confident individuals, ready to lead fulfilling lives as valued members of society.

Donaldson recommended that the curriculum be organised into:

- six "areas of learning and experience": expressive arts; health and wellbeing; humanities; languages, literacy and communication; maths and numeracy; and science and technology; and
- have three "cross-curriculum responsibilities" – literacy, numeracy and digital competence.

Further development of planning in this area, Welsh Government (2017) A new Curriculum for Wales, yields the following:

"Health and Wellbeing forms the foundation upon which a rounded and robust educational experience can be built both in terms of providing relevant skills and knowledge to promote healthy activities and practices... A set of key 'Themes' is required in order to organise the broad range of aspects of Health and Wellbeing. As a result, the following 6 indicative Thematic areas are defined; Personal Care and Development; Healthy Choices; Learning to Learn; Relationships and Emotions; Keeping Safe and Physical Activity."

Clearly there is much in the Donaldson report of relevance and value to the ideas being considered here.

In relation to the further and higher education agenda, the conclusions of the Hazelkorn (2016) review are of relevance. The principle of greater cooperation between the HE and FE sectors lies at the heart of the report, which should serve well the agenda under consideration here particularly in preparing a workforce which meets the needs of those wishing to study and learn in different and flexible ways as well as the needs of a healthcare system and its patients. As has been mentioned above, Health Education and Improvement Wales (HEIW), will have a leading role to play in achieving the goals being considered here.

How creative / innovative can we be?

It must be apparent that a step change in both culture and behaviour will likely be needed. A 'business as usual' model of delivery may not suffice i.e. doing more of the same will get more of the same and more of the same will not be what is needed in the future. Ideas that are more creative and innovative are needed. The 'Health and Care' sector does not exist in isolation. A creative / innovative response should, at least in theory, be driven by both the general economic pressures on the system, needs and the rapidly changing digital landscape. Strong and courageous leadership will also be needed.

The Bevan Commission, in its first report, A *Workforce Fit for the Future* (2016), states that "Bold and creative thinking and leadership will be required when planning ahead, trying out and combing new roles across a range of disciplines. More innovative ways to support people and the adoption of new skills are needed, such as; the use of IT and intergenerational skills programmes, using young people to support older people regards technology adoption."

The following skills will be key to any future health and care workforce and will need to be reflected in future training and development across the board.

- Analytical / problem solving skills – using data and other information to find the best solutions and ways of working e.g. using a range of data to inform and compare outcomes, achieve best value and monitor user feedback.

- Skills to use technology / IT – the ability to use IT and other forms of technology to help inform, support and connect the health and wellbeing of people e.g. use of home sensors and predictive technology.
- Communication / social skills – being able to communicate effectively with people will always be a core requirement and should not be taken for granted e.g. informed choice, choosing wisely and understanding need.

Creating the pace and scale for change

The recent Parliamentary Review (2018) into Health and Social Care in Wales called for "revolution not evolution" in the need to drive transformational change. The following provides further food for thought in the context of our education, skills and training environment and highlights some innovative and challenging opportunities:

- We need to create an ecosystem that focuses on health and wellbeing within our education systems, for our staff and for the pupils and students that we serve. We should do this by engaging and co-producing new innovative ideas and approaches with them drawing upon their ideas and initiatives along similar lines to the Bevan Innovators.
- We need to strongly develop the concept of a healthy Skills economy, to complement the work that has been carried out on the Knowledge economy.
- Techniques and the use of new technologies to support the development of new models of providing care should form a key part of the skills agenda.

- We need to consider a much greater role for apprenticeships in the Health and Care system. Other non-traditional forms of learning must be embraced including educating patients and using skills and wisdom of people who have recently retired and those who are returning to work after a period away.
- We should consider further the role of the Open University or an equivalent in the Health and Care system and the creation of a 'Health and Care' Digital Academy.
- We need to enable the skills and knowledge we already have to travel further, yielding greater cross pollination of disciplines to help solve problems e.g. computing and medicine or engineering and care.
- The Bevan Commission has already provided its advice on the need to move away from the traditional medical model of healthcare to a Social, Cooperative Model (Bevan Commission, 2017) which takes greater account of the wider impacts and solutions for health. It may also be that it is time to engage more closely with the further and higher education sector to consider how it might play a greater part in helping to determine, plan and deliver, in more innovative ways, skills that are fit and flexible to the future we have yet to fully understand.
- We need to develop better systems and mechanisms to ensure the effective transfer of knowledge and skills and ultimate adoption into practice. To achieve this, we need to encourage and incentivise adoption as well as development and innovation.

Conclusion

In conclusion, to change the way the future health and social care workforce is planned, trained and delivered will require a change in culture and ethos consistent with a prudent model of health as outlined by the Bevan Commission. We all have a role in NHS as citizens, as employers, as patients, as payers and as responsible members of society.

Acknowledgements

We are very grateful to Professor Keith Harding for his helpful advice and comments.

References

1. http://gov.wales/topics/health/nhswales/heiw/?lang=en

Bevan Commission (2015). Prudent Healthcare Principles paper

Bevan Commission (2016). *A workforce for prudent healthcare.*

Bevan Commission (2017). *A new way of thinking: A prudent model of health and care.*

Carers Wales (2018) available on line at https://www.carersuk.org/wales

Donaldson, G. (2015). *Successful Futures: Independent Review of Curriculum and Assessment Arrangements in Wales.*

Hazelkorn, E. (2016). *Towards 2030: A framework for building a world-class post-compulsory education system for Wales*

HEART (2017). The Health Enterprise Alliance for Regional Transformation, *A Strategic Blueprint for the Cardiff and Vale Health and Care System.*

The Parliamentary Review of Health and Social Care in Wales (2018) *A Revolution from Within.*

Welsh Government (2015). Well Being of Future Generations (Wales) Act

Welsh Government (2017). *A New curriculum for Wales*

17

Changing culture and capturing creativity of the Arts and Humanities to meet health needs across Wales

Professor John Wyn Owen

John has a career that has spanned public, private and charity sectors in the United Kingdom and internationally including the NHS, Civil Service, and Australia. He was the first Director of the NHS in Wales, Chair of the Secretary of State's Health Policy Board Executive Committee and Chair of the all Wales Health Services Authority. He has been Director General NSW State Health Ministry and Chair of the Australian Health Ministers Advisory Council and Secretary of the Nuffield Trust. Following retirement in 2005 held various positions: Chair, UWIC, Cardiff's Metropolitan University; Wales Board member and Chair of the Global Health Committee, Health Protection Agency; Chair Welsh Government's Health Protection Committee; Foundation Fellow and Treasurer Learned Society of Wales; Vice Chair UK Health Forum; Chair 2013 UK Canada Colloquium on New

Realities for Global Health; Senior Adviser Global Health Security InterAction Council; President, Johnians Society (Alumni), St John's College, Cambridge

Improving healthcare and wellbeing requires leadership that recognises the contribution of culture, arts, and the humanities in supporting the caring ambitions of every healthcare organisation and why we need a comprehensive health systems cultural barometer to measure progress in a multicultural Wales.

The arts and humanities touch people's lives at every level because they encompass those things that make lives worth living, contribute to a country's civilization and enhance the quality of health and wellbeing and help people cope with challenges of change. (Arts and Humanities Research Council)

In its Health 2020 strategy, WHO Europe expanded its definition of health, to include good health for communities as a resource that can contribute to achieving strong dynamic and creative societies and wellbeing resulting from a range of biomedical, psychological, social, economic and environmental factors that are interconnected across the life course.[1]

In 1998 the Nuffield Trust convened a conference to assess activities, perceptions, beliefs and models of effective practice of health professionals and the place of arts in both the community and healthcare environments to complement the scientific and technical models of diagnosis and treatment driving medical policies and practices in caring for people. The conference resolution 'The Windsor Declaration'[2] promoted the practical application of the arts as therapies, ethics and humanities in medical and health professional education and in public health and healthcare as well as community development for people of all backgrounds in prompting better health and wellbeing.

Following the declaration there was significant progress across the UK. In Wales, particularly noteworthy was the leadership for the elevated status of the medical humanities pioneered at Swansea University which created an unprecedented interdisciplinary post graduate study drawing together several interdisciplinary perspectives from the humanities and clinical medicine. Dr. David Greaves, co-director of the programme was also the founding editor of a new BMJ Journal Medical Humanities. The Welsh Government also recognised that there was connection between the arts and health and Edwina Hart, Health Minister stated, "People benefit from being in a conducive environment enhanced by good design and arts as well as from an active engagement in creative pursuits." Further, over the years, research in humanities and health has been well represented in Wales with major funding from Research Councils as well as support from the Welsh Arts Council.

In 2013 the Royal Society of Public Health convened a working group, chaired by the former secretary of the Nuffield Trust to review and report[3] on achievements since the Windsor Declaration as a contribution to an international conference on arts and culture for health and wellbeing. The report and his speech at the opening plenary of the international conference showed that the arts and health scene in the UK and internationally had changed dramatically, the economic crisis had created new realities for health globally and that market forces alone could not solve social problems and that greater equality had to become the new economic and social imperative with the arts and health and culture playing a crucial part in creating social capital for resilient individuals and communities.

In 2014, following the international conference, the UK Parliament established the All Party Parliamentary Group (APPG) on Arts Health and Well-being to improve awareness of the benefits that the arts can bring to health and wellbeing and to stimulate progress towards making these benefits a reality across the country. The National Assembly of Wales has also established a Cross Party Group for Arts and Health.

In 2017 the APPG, including evidence from Wales, published the results of an Inquiry with the view to making recommendations to improve policy and practice, including recognition that creativity can stimulate imagination and reflection; encourage dialogue with the deeper self and enable expression; change perspectives; increase control over life's circumstances; inspire change and growth as well as engender a sense of belonging and promote healing. Creativity was also seen as a means of empowerment that can help people to face problems.

The APPG report referenced Professor Crossick's in the AHRC cultural Value Project that "one of the most important things about health is self-reflection and empowerment and a sense that you can actually control what is damaging your health. This sense of mastery over one's environment leads to enhancement in health and wellbeing through the process of health creation."[4]

The APPG's Inquiry's conclusion was that the "UK is still very far from realizing more than a small modicum of the potential contribution of the arts to health and wellbeing and lag behind other countries such as Australia and the Nordic countries."[5] Further, that the arts could be enlisted to assist in addressing a number of difficult and pressing policy challenges: strengthening preventive strategies to maintain health for all; helping frail, and older people stay healthy and independent; enabling people to take a more active role in their own health and care; improving recovery from illness; enhancing mental health care; improving social care; mitigating social isolation and loneliness; strengthening local services and promoting more cohesive communities; enabling more cost effective use of resources within the NHS; increasing wellbeing amongst staff in health and social care; encouraging voluntary work; enhancing the quality of the built environment.

The APPG recognised however that the essential need is for cultural change; change in conventional thinking leading to change in conventional practice across complex systems of health and social care.

Nigel Crisp's book, *24 hours to save the NHS*[6], in which he claimed, "that systems thinking and leadership holds the key to many improvements in health and health care". The 'Cynefin' Framework[7], developed by David Snowdon, draws on research into complex adaptive systems theory, cognitive science, anthropology, and narrative patterns as well as evolutionary psychology to describe situations and systems. It explores relationships between people, experience, and context and proposes new approaches to communications, policy, decision-making and knowledge management in complex social environments.

The Cynefin Framework is ready made cultural change and there is an important opportunity for the arts health and wellbeing practitioners to be invited and contribute to the policy discussions on cultural competence for health systems - systems for health, health care and as learning systems - and smart governance. The Cynefin Framework has been adopted by the Victoria Health Department, Australia for health policy analysis, organisational strategy and for leading change.

Further the Cynefin Framework is related to place-based policy, a theme related to a British Academy (BA) Project "where we live now". The BA's project has been reviewing the evidence for people's attachments to place and the belief that places matter to people, they shape the way "we live our lives, feel ourselves and the relationships we have with others, memories and stories and our lived experience. All in turn contribute to personal and societal wellbeing." The view of the BA was that we "are surprisingly place blind when it comes to making policy for health, education, social care employment and the economy as if places were all the same." The WHO Euro Health 2020 calls for action across government and society for health and wellbeing to create resilient communities and supportive environments, to protect and promote health and a sense of belonging, what in Welsh we call Cynefin - a place where we instinctively belong or feel most connected.

Improving the quality healthcare and wellbeing not only requires systems but leadership, which recognises the contribution which culture - including arts and health - can make in supporting the caring ambitions of every health service organisation. Commenting on strategic management, leadership and organisational culture, Chris Edmunds (February 2013)[8] claimed: "...successful leaders when talking about their company or teams' performance light up about performance metrics but don't when they talk about organisational culture; but those that do, understand that organisation's culture is one of their most important assets. The reality is that most leaders do not have measuring or monitoring systems that keep them informed about the quality of their organisation's culture and the advice to business is to make culture as important as performance."

UK health managers might want to explore US experience in health management education and the place of culture in academic programmes. At the AUPHA 2013 Annual Meeting (American Association of Programs Health Administration) there was a session on how to teach cultural competence on undergraduate and graduate programmes with particular attention to provide sensitivity, cultural based healing, cultural concordance, cultural proficiency competency and awareness in the world of healthcare administration.

Challenges of cultural competence were identified by the Francis Inquiry and called for action so that every single person serving patients contribute to a compassionate caring service and recommended a shared culture and that a "tool or methodology such as a cultural barometer to measure the cultural health of all parts of the system". A somewhat limited interpretation internal to health service institutions has been put on this recommendation, interpreting the recommendation as restricted to matters of values, standards, safety, honesty and transparency. There is a need for more comprehensive metrics for health services and culture (including arts and humanities and health) beyond simply the internal health care organisation to create a fully comprehensive health systems cultural barometer of resilient individuals, communities, institutions and healthcare organisations. In short, defining the way of life of a society and health in line with the ONS initiative on measuring what matters and understanding the Nations wellbeing.

This contribution (to the Bevan Commission's NHS@70) has focused on new realities for health and the contribution of the arts, humanities and culture for individual and community resilience - key elements in the Well-being of

Future Generations (Wales) Act 2015 and commends the policy recommendations of the APPG to the Welsh Government to encourage an up-scaling of joint activities by the Arts Council and Health Boards in complementing and enhancing the effectiveness of conventional medicine.

Times of continuing economic vulnerability require governments to take action and enable long needed but politically challenging reforms such as "shaping the boundaries of the state of the future"[9]. Business as usual is not an option and a transformative shift is essential to cope with life's uncertainties, the need for more social inclusion, new solutions, and good governance in the changing roles of the citizen and the state and wellbeing.

Ways forward would be for the Government of Wales with the NHS@70 to:

1.   Press for health smart investments in culture, humanities, and the arts with economic and other benefits that will protect, promote, and improve the health and wellbeing of the people of Wales.

2.   Health leaders in Wales, - national, regional and local - must press for and implement health policy interventions which promote social capital, individual and community resilience by drawing on the work of the APPG and the Welsh Assembly's Cross Party Arts and Health, in particular health impact assessment of all policies including culture and the arts and health - arts as therapies, in community development and health and humanities in health professional education.

3.   The arts and health communities in Wales - practitioners and academics - need to come together to create national and regional networks (Forums) to build on the work of the cross-party group of the National Assembly and the Welsh Arts Council to renew a strategic direction for culture, arts health and wellbeing in Wales and to provide evidence and guidance in keeping with the ambitions of the Wellbeing of Future Generations Act (Wales) 2015.

4. Ensure a better culture of health and wellbeing, by supporting the caring ambitions of every health service organisation and investing in research and education and professional development.

After all the Windsor Declaration of 1998[2] emphasised that "change must accept that Britain, is a society of many races, cultures, religions and habits and health professionals and health systems must be aware of the need to understand such diversity, to learn how to communicate with persons of whatever background and be prepared to initiate, adapt and comprehend change."

A comprehensive cultural barometer of the health system - the resilience of individuals, communities, institutions, and healthcare organisations - would tell us whether we are making progress towards a culture of better health and wellbeing for all in Wales.

References

1. WHO Regional Office for Europe (2013) *Health 2020 A European policy framework and strategy for the 21st Century.* Copenhagen.
2. Phillip, R., Baum, M., Mawson A., Calman, Sir K., 1999 *Humanities in Medicine: Beyond the Millennium. A summary of the proceedings of the first Windsor Conference.* Nuffield Trust Series No 10.
3. *Arts Health and Wellbeing Beyond the Millennium; how far have we come and where do want to go?* RSPH Working Group Report published by the RSPH and Phillip Family Foundation 2013.
4. Crossick, G. & Kaszynska, P., (2016) *Understanding the Value of Arts and Culture: The AHRC Cultural Value Project.* AHRC Swindon.
5. APPG Arts and Health Inquiry Report July 2017.
6. Crisp, N., *24 Hours to Save the NHS. The Chief Executive's Account of reform 2000-2006,* Oxford University Press 2011.
7. David J., Snowden, Mary E., Boone. A. *Leaders Framework for Decision Making.* Harvard Business Review, 2007.
8. Edmunds, C. *Your Organizational Culture Probably Needs Tending. Smart Brief on Leadership: Innovative Ideas Ahead of the Curve.* Smart Brief Inc. Washington DC .27 February 2013.
9. *Shaping boundaries of the State.* Financial Times 4. December 2015.

18

Why are voluntary organisations feeling it is getting harder to engage with the NHS?

Sir Paul Williams OBE KStJ DL

Sir Paul's career in the NHS spanned forty-five years where he was the Chief Executive of three NHS Trusts and President of the Institute of Healthcare Management. His final job was Director General for Health and Social Services, Welsh Assembly Government and CEO, NHS Wales. He is a non-executive director of Natural Resources Wales and Chair of the People and Remuneration Committee and Chair of the Public Transport Users Advisory Panel. He is a Trustee and Board Member, Royal Voluntary Service and Chair of the Investment Committee, Trustee and Chair of the Royal Masonic Benevolent Institution Care Company and Trustee for the Masonic Charitable Foundation and a Visiting Professor at the University of South Wales.

Voluntary organisations are claiming it is getting harder to engage and develop mutually beneficial partnerships with the NHS at a time when pressure and demand on the Health Service is at an all-time high.

This year the NHS celebrates its 70th Anniversary and intends to recognise the important role the voluntary sector plays. Will 2018 mark an important turning point, or just a brief pause in a drifting relationship?

If indeed the claims of a number of voluntary organisations are correct, is this a symptom of an NHS under stress and turning within itself as it struggles to achieve targets? Or is it both the health and third sector feeling the pressures after 10 years of austerity? Are there other factors at work which need to be understood and addressed which could lead to a better appreciation of the complimentary roles of the statutory and third sector? Indeed, would a strengthening of these complimentary roles lead to a more sustainable future for both?

Over the last 10 years the Bevan Commission has been developing the concept of prudent healthcare as a means of tackling today's challenges whilst remaining true to Aneurin Bevan's founding principles. What would Bevan have made of a health service where the voluntary sector feels less valued? Well first it has to be said Aneurin Bevan's battles to form the NHS were not just with the BMA and the influential teaching hospitals. Over a quarter of the hospital beds he proposed to nationalise were run by voluntary organisations who expressed concerns about a loss of local control. To accommodate these concerns voluntary organisations were represented on local hospital management committees. This strengthened grass roots support and helped channel additional resources – money and volunteers – into and expanding and infant NHS. This special relationship prospered in the first half century of the NHS. In NHS Wales this link remains and in last reorganisation in 2009/10, a non-officer member representing the voluntary sector was included in the constitution of the new Local Health Boards. However, in evidence given by representatives of the voluntary sector in the Parliamentary Review of NHS Wales, some expressed concerns of a lack of engagement despite having representation on Local Health Boards.

In the early 70s most health authorities in Wales employed full time voluntary service coordinators as a means of maximising the ties between the NHS and the voluntary sector. Almost all hospitals of any size (or groups of hospitals) had a thriving League of Friends which raised money and provided support for their hospital from the local community. The voluntary sector was seen as an important and vital source of funding and providing a range of valued volunteers. Their prominent role made them influential stakeholders in the provision of local services.

I well remember my first CEO position with the Bridgend and District NHS Trust where the WRVS and Red Cross ran the hospital reception desks, shops, tea bars, trolley services and the League of Friends raised substantial sums of money for patient comforts through to equipment and building upgrades. Specialist charities like Macmillan provided a much-needed local hospice and the generosity of the public supported by numerous local charities funded the first CT Scanner. This partnership was replicated across the NHS at the time. The role played by the voluntary sector in the so-called priority services (what a misnomer) channelling funds into services for the elderly, mental health, learning disabilities and substance misuse. The voluntary sector played a key role in pioneering new approaches to service delivery which were innovative and accessible, often where the statutory sector was slow to evolve and held back by red tape. The millions flowing into research, cancer care and other specialist areas clearly have to be acknowledged.

Today according to the Charity Commission the Sector is worth £70 bn and with over 160,000 organisations. Recent research by the WCVA suggests that in Wales across the whole sector there are some 30,000 organisations, 938,000 volunteers at a value of £3.8 bn. Clearly this is not all health related but demonstrates the size of the sector. However, a point which will be made later which is worth trailing here, is the incalculable health and wellbeing benefits of over 900,000 people in Wales being engaged in meaningful activity.

Given the size and influence of the voluntary sector, why is there an apparent drift away from a previously strong and mutually beneficial relationship with the NHS? First it should be said that, if this is indeed the case, the fault may not entirely be placed at the door of the NHS. However, this may be a good place to start and ironically for the best of reasons. The Blair Government's commitment to substantially increase the funding to the NHS may have caused it to be less reliant on seeking the support from charities and the voluntary sector. This may in turn over time have led to a loss of corporate memory of how important the third sector formally was and how to maintain and foster strong links. The PFI programme in England certainly hit organisations like the RVS hard who lost out to high street chains when in competition for retail space in new hospital developments. Facilities Managers may have extracted the maximum income from the floor area rented out, but the Trust or Health Board has lost out on gifting ploughed back by charities like RVS, together with the compassionate ear of volunteers for patients and staff and not to minimise the benefit to the community of having an active group of volunteers.

The increasing role of Regulators and burden of legislation has put pressure on the third sector to become more 'professional' which often impacted on the traditional volunteers who needed to change in order comply with new governance requirements.

As austerity began to bite, grants from the statutory sector began to dry up. This reduced the interface / engagement between the NHS and third sector. The loss of grant income also required the voluntary sector to search for new income streams turning to providing a range of commercial services often filling an essential gap following the withdrawal by the statutory sector. In recent years, many have become very adept in this new role, but in doing so have opened themselves up to criticism of diluting their core charitable purpose and undervaluing their own volunteers in favour of a paid workforce. Another unintended consequence may have been to put themselves in direct competition with parts of the NHS as commercial operators who could threaten NHS jobs rather than be seen as a trusted partner supplementing essential work.

In this rapidly changing world, charities are no longer the only organisations involved in this area, so the NHS has also to consider and engage community interest companies and social enterprises which are also filling the space which was the province of the voluntary sector. Some voluntary organisations have found it difficult to adapt to a business model where grants no longer exist or are hard to obtain. Trust may be another factor with media concerns about fund raising practices, CEO salaries and poor governance all hitting the headlines.

These few examples suggest that there are many factors at work here which need to be identified and understood. The role of the voluntary sector in today's NHS may have not received the attention of policy makers to the degree to which it should, given the size and rich diversity of the sector. The Welsh Government report, Designed to Add Value in Wales, was published in 2008 and was perhaps the last major publication to last to focus on this important area in some depth. This lack of focus seems strange given the current and predicted challenges facing NHS Wales. Very few if any delivery plans give much consideration of the significant opportunities which exist to develop the relationship. However, in England, this may well change following the setting up in 2017 of Helpforce, a community interest company which aims to enable volunteering to play a greater role in supporting NHS staff. Helpforce believe well managed staff and volunteer teams can make an important contribution to improving patient care in hospitals. As workforce issues are likely to be the dominant factor in defining the future shape and capacity of the NHS, policy makers would do well to follow the progress of the Helpforce initiative.

The role of the voluntary sector is hardly peripheral and ranges from raising hard cash for donations, purchase of equipment, new buildings etc. to:

- Supporting research and leading edge thinking;
- Operating commercial services;
- Offering expertise and advice;
- Sponsoring new partners;
- Being innovative, transformational, responsive and flexible;
- A beacon for disadvantaged groups;

- Providing user friendly and bespoke services for particularly hard to reach client groups;
- Prepare young people for the world of work;
- Promote community resilience and cohesion;
- Supplement a traditional workforce model; and
- Bestow the benefits of health and wellbeing on those that volunteer – over 900,000 in Wales.

This list is far from complete but surely raises the serious question of how much added value the NHS is missing by not engaging as fully as possible with the voluntary sector? Some Welsh Health Boards do work hard to develop their links with the voluntary sector and employ coordinators but the situation is mixed with some being financed from charitable funds and others on short term contracts. Whilst these efforts are to be commended they may lack a strategic approach warranted to match the breadth and scale of services provided by Health Boards and indeed the increasing number of charities and voluntary organisations. Indeed, are Health Boards in Wales certain they know the extent of the potential added value the voluntary sector and charities could bring to over stretched services in their area? Are they prioritising sufficient time and resources to maximise the huge potential added value and making full use of their voluntary sector non-officer members?

The first principle of Prudent Healthcare is:

> *'Achieve health and well-being with the public,*
> *patients and professionals as equal partners*
> *through co- production.'*

Let's not miss the opportunity of the 70th anniversary of the NHS and recognising the role of the voluntary sector to rekindle this special relationship.

19

Addressing health inequalities in Wales

Professor Sir Michael Marmot
MBBS MPH PhD FRCP FFPHM FMedSci FBA

Sir Michael is Professor of Epidemiology at University College London, and Immediate Past President of the World Medical Association. He has led research groups on health inequalities for 40 years. He chairs the Commission on Equity and Health Inequalities in the Americas and was Chair of the Commission on Social Determinants of Health (CSDH), which was set up by the World Health Organization in 2005, and produced the report entitled: 'Closing the Gap in a Generation' in August 2008. At the request of the British Government, he conducted the Strategic Review of Health Inequalities in England post 2010, which published its report 'Fair Society, Healthy Lives' in February 2010. This was followed by the European Review of Social Determinants of Health and the Health Divide, for WHO Euro in 2014. He served as President of the British Medical Association (BMA) in 2010-2011, and is President of the British

Lung Foundation. He is an Honorary Fellow of the American College of Epidemiology; a Fellow of the Academy of Medical Sciences; an Honorary Fellow of the British Academy, and an Honorary Fellow of the Faculty of Public Health of the Royal College of Physicians and is a member of the National Academy of Medicine.

It is good news that for Wales, more people are expected to live longer, and indeed the population of 75s and over is projected to increase by 50% between 2014 and 2030 (Welsh Government, 2016). There are however two important points to note, firstly – life expectancy has not been increasing as quickly in Wales as it has in England, and secondly, along with the rest of the UK, there are marked health inequalities, with approximately a 10-year gap between the life expectancy of those living in deprived and those living in less deprived areas in some areas in Cardiff. This is not just a social injustice, but health inequalities are also estimated to cost £3-4 billion annually through higher welfare payments, productivity losses, lost taxes and additional illness (Welsh Assembly Government, 2011).

A focus on life expectancy only presents some of the picture, and tends to place our focus on older people. At the other end of the spectrum, health indicators for children show similar trends, for example childhood obesity varies between most and least deprived communities. Some 28.4% of children living in the most deprived areas are either overweight or obese compared to 20.9% in the least deprived areas (Public Health Wales, 2017). Twice as many children living in Merthyr Tydfil, for example, are obese compared to those living in the Vale of Glamorgan (14.7% Merthyr Tydfil, 7.3% Vale of Glamorgan). Instances of childhood injuries and tooth decay show similar patterns (Public Health Wales Observatory, 2017a).

Although infant mortality rates have declined in recent years in Wales, neonatal and infant mortality rates are still highest in the most deprived areas of the country, almost 50% more than in the least deprived areas. Children living in the most deprived areas are twice as likely to be of low birth weight and half as likely to be breast fed compared to children in the least deprived areas (Public Health Wales Observatory, 2017b).

Recent research from Public Health Wales (2016a) has also highlighted the lifelong impacts of adverse childhood experiences (ACEs) such as physical, domestic and sexual abuse. Exposure of young children to adverse experiences, in the first two to three years of life when the brain is rapidly developing, can set individuals on a life course of disadvantage and anti-social and possibly violent behaviour. The Healthy Child Wales Programme was introduced in 2016 in response and to provide universal support to all families during the first 1,000 days of a child's life as well as targeted support to high risk families.

Addressing health inequalities, from birth, and throughout the life-course is essential.

Local and national action needed to address the social determinants of health

Addressing health inequalities in Wales needs a combination of evidence-based politics and a spirit of social justice, invoking the legacy of Aneurin Bevan. The Marmot review undertaken at the Institute of Health Equity (IHE) identified six policy objectives (Marmot, 2010):

- Give every child the best start in life.
- Enable all children, young people and adults to maximise their capabilities and have control over their lives.
- Create fair employment and good work for all.
- Ensure a healthy standard of living for all.
- Create and develop healthy and sustainable places and communities.
- Strengthen the role and impact of ill health prevention.

Public Health Wales (2016b) has set out a related array of mechanisms to reduce ill health and inequalities. While there is more of a focus on behaviour here there is the clear recognition of the need to reduce poverty.

- Ensuring a good start in life for all.
- Promoting mental wellbeing and preventing mental ill health.
- Preventing violence and abuse.
- Reducing prevalence of smoking.
- Reducing prevalence of alcohol misuse.
- Promoting physical activity.
- Promoting healthy diet and preventing obesity.
- Protection from disease and early identification.
- Reducing economic and social inequalities and mitigating austerity.
- Ensuring a safe and health-promoting natural and built environment.

The policy objectives are clearly not all within the traditional remit of government health ministries. To achieve success and move forward, combined action with buy in across government departments is required. It is therefore extremely encouraging to note that the Welsh Government is at the forefront of thinking regarding this. Two landmark Welsh laws have recently been passed. The Social Services and Well-being (Wales) Act 2014 and the Wellbeing of Future Generations (Wales) Act 2015 require public bodies to work together for the long-term sustainability of Wales and its people. This includes the NHS which is the largest employer in Wales and is responsible for the largest area of spend for the Welsh Government (Welsh Government, 2016).

The Social Services and Well-being Act aims to improve health and wellbeing by modernising the law regarding social care. The Act aims to give people greater control over the care and support they receive. Similar to public health provision in England, there is a focus on population needs assessment, preventative services, information provision, partnership working and an expectation that care will be integrated. It is intended that the NHS in Wales is will work collaboratively with other agencies to deliver health and wellbeing gains for the population.

Connected to this is the Well-being of Future Generations (Wales) Act which provides a new framework to address inequalities. In a similar vein, it also sets out expectations for partnership working among public bodies including the NHS as well as creating an individual duty for some statutory organisations to contribute to a series of wellbeing goals.

In addition, central to making change are local authorities and committed leaders. Not all action necessarily requires central government mandate, and local areas with increasing freedom over budgets can also be the agents of effective change. Local individuals may also drive positive change through community interest companies. These can be used to set up local sports clubs or health and wellbeing groups which increase people's connectedness and access to physical activity.

Moving on from the Marmot review – change is possible.

Central to this chapter, is a message that IHE are keen to convey – change is possible.

Since the review in 2010, IHE have continued to build the evidence base on health inequalities, and driven by demand, have written a number of reports to aid implementation of these recommendations. Central to this work was a strong commitment from public health officials to improve the social determinants of health, both nationally in the health agencies, and locally. However, officials were not sure how they would actually achieve better early years outcomes, or better quality of work, for example. For Public Health England, a number of publications were written to aid local area officials to forward recommendations, with examples of best practice. In addition, work with the medical and allied health professions has helped to identify their role and monitoring of the social determinants at a local area level has helped to inform on progress.

Figure 1 - % of children attaining 5+ GCSEs and inequality gap 2014/15

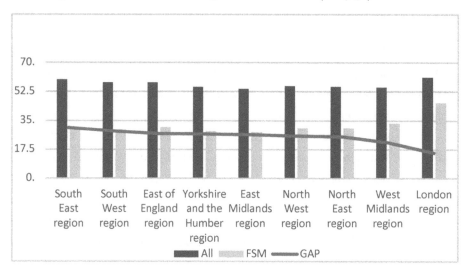

One example is from our annual indicator work, and relates to reducing the gap in attainment between the general population of children and those eligible for free school meals. Figure 1 illustrates a sizeable gap in attainment between those on free school meals and all across the country. However, take a look at the bars for London on the right. In London, children from poorer families do much better than in the rest of the country, and at no detriment to the general figures. Roll out of effective strategies, and analytical work to understand these differences is warranted, however the fundamental point is... look! You can narrow the gap between all children and those that are on free school meals, because it has already been done.

The annual indicator work that we conduct monitors progress across all areas on each of the policy objectives, and it is clear that there are some areas, for each indicator, that given a certain level of deprivation are doing better than expected. For example, we also looked at the best and worst performers in terms of the gap in attainment at age 5 between all and those who would be eligible for a free school meal. On average in England there is a 15.6 percentage point difference, but in Hackney, it is only a 4.2 percentage point difference, whereas in Bath and Somerset, it is nearly a 30 percentage point difference. Clearly Hackney is doing something right. Spreading best practice from the better performing areas should be a key policy priority.

Another example relates to secondary analyses of life expectancy figures over time, and finds – despite perhaps a general sense that government policies have not managed to improve health inequalities – quite the opposite. Over the period 2004 - 2012, explicit targets were in place to reduce the gap in life expectancy and infant mortality between the most and least deprived. During the time of the strategy the life expectancy gap between the most and the least deprived areas began to reduce, but these gaps increased prior to the strategy and after. Some of this success has been attributed to the success of Spearhead areas, and policy makers might wish to learn from this example.

The English government did not take on all the recommendations from the Marmot review, and was famously silent on the issue of having a minimum income for healthy living. The latest indicators for this, based on Joseph Rowntree Foundation data (JRF, 2018) suggest that the numbers on insufficient incomes have been increasing. Evidence from the EU Statistics on Income and Living Conditions (EU-Silc) illustrates that material deprivation is a strong predictor of self-reported ill health, much more so than income itself or education (WHO, 2014). Ensuring that people have sufficient income to be healthy should be a policy priority led by central government, not least because insufficient income will transfer to greater costs to the health services at a later stage. We know that in Sweden levels of material deprivation are the lowest in Europe, unsurprising therefore that they have small inequalities in health compared to the UK. Local areas may struggle to counter economic austerity, but might want to push through a requirement to pay the real living wage in public bodies, and their contracts following the example of Islington for example, and might try to incentivise local private employers to do the same.

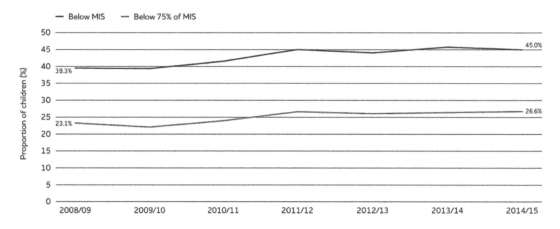

Figure 2 – Percentage of children below MIS and below 75% of MIS

Source: JRF (2015) Households below a Minimum Income Standard: 2008/09 to 2014/15

In addition to these broad examples, IHE have identified, for various areas, a number of best practice interventions. For example, for a report that we are currently writing that applies a social determinants approach to people with learning difficulties, we have found that work outcomes could be increased by 45 percentage points if a successful supported employment programme was introduced, and negative parenting behaviour to children with learning difficulties could be reduced by 40 percentage points.

In the Public Health England (PHE) 'Addressing health inequalities at a local level' series, we provide examples and links on a range of topics, from parenting interventions to improving the quality of work, from school transition processes to healthy high streets. There are plenty of examples to draw from, the key is to ensure that the best interventions are chosen for a particular area.

The medical and health profession moving forward

The development of local (and national) action plans based on a combination of local needs assessment, asset and policy mapping, and the identification of effective strategies and interventions is something that health professionals can take a lead in. In addition, doctors can work for health equity through international medical associations such as the World Medical Association and national medical associations.

Health professionals have an important and often under-utilised role in reducing health inequalities (Institute of Health Equity, 2013). The health workforce is well placed to develop services that impact on the wider social determinants of health and reduce inequities through:

- Workforce education and training;
- Practical actions to be taken during interactions with patients;
- Ways of working in Partnership; and
- advocacy.

Given that illness arises from the conditions in which people are born, grow, live, work, and age – the social determinants of health – it's clear that all agencies have a role in reducing the causes of illness and, indeed, the causes of the causes. Action on the social determinants of health should be a core part of health professionals' business, as it improves clinical outcomes, and saves money and time in the longer term. But, most persuasively, taking action to reduce health inequalities is a matter of social justice and all sectors of society have a role in reducing inequalities.

A call to action

Social injustice is killing on a grand scale. We know that improved health equity can be delivered through action on the social determinants of health by taking a life course approach and following best practice that is already available. Of course, there is always room for improvement and new initiatives should be encouraged and evaluated, but there is the possibility with what we know now to positively change outcomes, now.

References

Institute of Health Equity (2013). *Working for Health Equity: The Role of Health Professionals.* http://www.instituteofhealthequity.org/resources-reports/working-for-health-equity-the-role-of-health-professionals. (Accessed 30 April 2018)

Joseph Rowntree Foundation (JRF) (2018). *UK Poverty Data* https://www.jrf.org.uk/data (Accessed 30 April 2018)

Joseph Rowntree Foundation (JRF) (2015). *Households below a minimum income standard.* https://www.jrf.org.uk/report/households-below-minimum-income-standard-200809-201415. (Accessed 22 May 2018)

Marmot, M. et al., (2010) *Fair Society Healthy Lives (The Marmot Review).* London: Institute of Health Equity. http://www.instituteofhealthequity.org/resources-reports/fair-society-healthy-lives-the-marmot-review

Mental Health Foundation (2016). *Mental Health in Wales. Fundamental Facts in 2016.* https://www.mentalhealth.org.uk/sites/default/files/FF16%20Wales.pdf (Accessed 20 April 2018)

NHS Wales Shared Services Partnership (2018). http://www.nwssp.wales.nhs.uk/home. (Accessed 22 April 2018]

Olatunde O. (2015). *Life Expectancy at Birth and at Age 65 by Local Areas in England and Wales: 2012 to 2014* [Internet]. Office for National Statistics; 2015 p.4. Available from: http://www.ons.gov.uk/peoplepopulationandcommunity/birthsdeathsandmarriages/lifeexpectancies/bulletins/ lifeexpectancyatbirthandatage65bylocalareasinenglandandwales/. (Accessed 22 April 2018]

ONS (2017) Population Estimates for UK, England and Wales, Scotland and Northern Ireland – Office for National Statistics [Internet]. Available from: www.ons.gov.uk/peoplepopulationandcommunity/populationandmigration/populationestimates/datasets/populationestimatesforukenglandandwalesscotlandandnorthernireland. (Accessed 20 April 2018)

Public Health Wales (2016a). *Adverse Childhood Experiences and their impact on health-harming behaviours in the Welsh adult population.* http://www.wales.nhs.uk/sitesplus/888/news/40000/ (Accessed 30 April 2018)

Public Health Wales (2016b). *Making a Difference: Investing in Sustainable Health and Well-being for the People of Wales* [Internet]. 2016. Available from: http://www.wales.nhs.uk/sitesplus/888/page/87106. (Accessed 22 April 2018)

Public Health Wales (2017). *The Child Measurement Programme for Wales 2015/16.* http://www.wales.nhs.uk/sitesplus/documents/888/12518%20PHW%20CMP%20Report%20%28Eng%29.pdf. (Accessed 20 April 2018)

Public Health Wales Observatory (2017a). *Public Health Outcomes Framework using Welsh Dental Survey (WOHIU) and WIMD 2014 (WG)* [Internet]. 2017. Available from: https://public.tableau.com/profile/ publichealthwalesobservatory#!/vizhome/shared/FRNFQR5DR

Public Health Wales Observatory (2017b). *Public Health Outcomes Framework using NCCHD (NWIS) and WIMD 2014 (WG)* [Internet]. 2017. Available from: https://public.tableau.com/profile/publichealthwalesobservatory#!/vizhome/shared/WB8BMZZ5Q

Stats Wales (2017). https://statswales.gov.wales/Catalogue. (Accessed 23 April 2018)

Together for Health (2015). Respiratory Annual Report 2015 http://www.wales.nhs.uk/documents/27724_English%20Combined%20WEB.PDF. (Accessed 22 April 2018)

Welsh Assembly Government (2011). *Fairer Health Outcomes for All.* http://www.wales.nhs.uk/sitesplus/documents/866/5.1%20Appendix%20Fairer%20Outcomes%20for%20All-Welsh%20Assembly%20Government%20Document.pdf. (Accessed 23 April 2018)

Welsh Government (2015). http://www.legislation.gov.uk/anaw/2015/2/contents/enacted. (Accessed 30 April 2018)

Welsh Government (2016). *Local Authority Population Projections for Wales (2014-based): Principal projection* [Internet]. 2016 p.11. http://gov.wales/statistics-and-research/local-authority-population-projections/?lang=en. (Accessed 22 April 2018)

Welsh Government (2016). *Rebalancing Health Care.* http://gov.wales/docs/dhss/publications/161110cmoreport16en.pdf (Accessed 30 April 2018)

Welsh Government (2017a). *Future Trends Report 2017*, p5. http://gov.wales/statistics-and-research/future-trends/?lang=en. (Accessed 22 April 2018)

Welsh Government (2017b) *National Survey for Wales.* http://gov.wales/statistics-and-research/national-survey/?lang=en. (Accessed 23 April 2018)

Welsh Government (2017c). *Gambling with our Health* http://gov.wales/docs/phhs/publications/cmo-report2017en.pdf. (Accessed 20 April 2017)

Welsh Health Survey (2014-15) http://gov.wales/statistics-and-research/welsh-health-survey/?lang=en. (Accessed 22 April 2018)

World Health Organisation (WHO) 2014. *Review of social determinants and the health divide in the WHO European Region: final report.* http://www.euro.who.int/__data/assets/pdf_file/0004/251878/Review-of-social-determinants-and-the-health-divide-in-the-WHO-European-Region-FINAL-REPORT.pdf. (Accessed 30 April 2018)

20

Making this all work in practice

Professor Sir Mansel Aylward CB
Helen Howson

This book marks 10 years of the achievements of Bevan Commission as well as celebrating the 70th Anniversary of the NHS. It brings together the personal reflections and views of the Bevan Commissioners, as internationally acclaimed experts in their respective fields. They use the Social Model for Health and Care as a basis to discuss how sustaining health and care starts with people and in communities, how innovation can transform services and how there is still much work to be done to tackle health inequality and apply the changes needed at speed. Together these represent the collective thinking of the Bevan Commissioners, their wisdom, experience and foresight alongside practical solutions for many of the problems that we face both here in Wales and further afield.

These build upon the key achievements of the Bevan Commission, most notably the concept of Prudent Healthcare and more recently the Social Model of Health. The Commission recognised the unsustainability of the current system which predominantly treats ill health at the expense of promoting health and wellbeing.

In response, it proposed a different model of health and care for Wales, one that is not just based upon fixing people in the traditional way, but one which applies the four prudent principles to preventing and protecting health and treating ill health most effectively using all skills and resources to best effect. It recognises that individual and collective health is everyone's responsibility; it cannot be just the responsibility of the NHS.

We believe this concept, together with the views expressed within the book, makes a powerful and compelling case for change, which the Bevan Commission will continue to champion. The role the Commission plays as an independent, authoritative voice that can both advise and act as a critical friend to support and promote change is crucial to this success.

The future of health and care is not bright unless we address the impending manpower crisis which may see a shortfall of 14.5 million medical professionals by 2030 (WHO, 2013). Over the next 70 years, alongside developing a globally competitive workforce, we must recruit the population as allies and willing partners, recognising their needs which includes self-care, family care, and care by community. This will enable the NHS to adapt to radical changes and deploy its professionals in new and innovative ways, recognising that the State cannot provide everything.

In the translation of its thinking into practice, driving and supporting such change, the Bevan Commission Academy has played a key role. The Bevan Innovators, Exemplars, Advocates and Fellows have all played a key part. The breadth and range of projects alongside the inspiration and enthusiasm shown by participants is truly inspiring. It clearly demonstrates how people, communities and professionals can, with a little help, change the way they think and operate, identifying innovative ideas to meet the challenges and needs we face.

Health and care services will need to be more focused upon people's needs, not just on paper but in reality. We must find better ways in which we can re-design services around needs together and not vice versa without being constrained by existing roles and responsibilities. The future workforce will need to be flexible and responsive to change much of which we have yet to realise. We will need to be better at using all the skills and resources we have available to us, whether in health or social care, as patients or professionals or with other partners such as industry and the third sector. It is imperative that we come together to find the solutions to make this work in reality.

The people of Wales will need to work with us as key partners in this journey. By working together, they will help translate prudence into practice, being actively involved in determining their own health, wellbeing and care and in fashioning a Welsh cooperative, national health and care service which soundly meet their needs and those of others in the future. From birth to end of life we will need their input and insight to achieve the desired future.

The international community will continue to observe and learn from us in Wales in maintaining a sustainable, universal, comprehensive and affordable national health and care service for its people. It shall endure and blossom, as it has during its last 70 years, responding to challenge and change for the next 70 years to come. The Bevan Commission will work with its people to ensure it continues to be the cherished legacy left to us by the architect of the NHS, Aneurin Bevan, in the way he intended.